PARENTING STYLES

Dr. Smritikana Ghosh

The Pustakalaya

The Pustakalaya
Near Indian Bank, Old Jail Road
Bangla Bazar, Lucknow - 226002
Email - thepustakalaya.in@gmail.com

First Published in 2023

Parenting Styles

First Edition 2023
Educational Psychology | 9789391900021

Editing- Dr. Smritikana Ghosh
Book Formatting & Cover Design- Shubham Singh
(The Pustakalaya)

CONTENTS

CHAPTER-1

INTRODUCTION

The functioning of society is dependent on the institution of the family, which not only has a substantial bearing on the human condition but also plays an important part in social life. There is little questioning that families have a significant impact on society; yet, determining the extent of that impact may be exceedingly challenging. Lifelong effects of adverse childhood events are well-documented. An individual's survival and flourishing depend on the solid ground provided by their parents. Children need the love and care of their parents and cannot be raised in isolation. Although if they are vulnerable to the impacts of society and culture, the family nevertheless plays a significant part in the formation of their thoughts and attitudes. According to the findings of this research, families have a significant influence on the education that their children get, particularly in the areas of creativity, physical development, and moral development. The majority of parents place a high importance on having a right and healthy relationship with their children, and this is one of the many elements that influence their children's mental and physical welfare. According to a body of research, the level of communication that exists between parents and their offspring is one of the most important factors in shaping a child's personality. The relationship between a parent and a kid may exist for a variety of reasons, including the need to ensure the child's existence, to provide comfort and love, to foster communication, to encourage the child, to provide for the child, and to enforce rules.

Pupils are provided with the opportunities to acquire skills such as being familiar with the norms and practices of the society from the viewpoint of their parents, in addition to the other educational goals of teaching morality and ethics, values, and emotional literacy. Being a mother is one of the first difficulties that a parent looks forward to successfully overcoming, despite the fact that it may be rather difficult. Families are crucial in respect to child growth, and so are parental behaviours in regard to child social and emotional development. This is true in much the same way as other social and educational environments are significant. Because a parent is someone who lives up to the expectations of a family and someone who serves as a positive role model in the community, parenting frequently determines how a family and a community act towards one another. Without parents to teach their children about appropriate behaviour, there would be no such thing as a family or a civilised society. It is essential for parents and adolescents to work together because this collaboration helps mould adolescents' perspectives by modifying and controlling their relationships with the influences of other family members, in addition to having an impact that is beyond the control of the family alone. When it comes to adolescence, the most significant impact that a person's parents may have on their lives is the effect that they have. Parents are a child's first and most influential instructors. A large portion of a child's development will depend on their relationship with their parents. Hence, parents should tailor their approach to raising their kid such that it brings out the best in him or her. How you discipline and care for your child will have a significant impact on how they turn out. Parental effects are the most important in shaping adolescent behavior, and it is often believed that these affects are more pervasive than in the teenagers' actual social environment. Adolescents, it is generally agreed, need to establish stable, loving relationships with adults in order to thrive emotionally and psychologically. This is why many people believe it is crucial for adolescents to grow up in loving, nurturing homes. Permissive parents are those who are prepared to wait on their children, make few demands of them, and who push their kids to talk about their emotions and act on their impulses with few repercussions. The use of shame and the threat of severe emotional deprivation via inactivity as a form of punishment for children are, to some extent, consistent with permissive parenting's message that getting one's way by manipulating others is acceptable. Children from dysfunctional families tend to be narcissistic or have narcissistic tendencies themselves, as well as act impulsively and self-centeredly in social interactions.

Concept of Parenting

Indian parents often take up the major role of child careers in the home. Inasmuch as most children rely on their parents for everything from sustenance and safety to financial support and emotional support, it seems to reason that parents would hold the position of greatest influence in their lives. Parenting is a method of bringing up children in which the father and mother take turns, or work together, to help their offspring become productive members of society and culture who may later use these experiences to help them feel a sense of belonging and stability. The responsibilities that parents play in their children's passage from childhood to adulthood have become more important. Parenthood has been regarded as a primary mechanism in socializing the kid. The term "parenting" refers to the act of becoming a parent as well as the process of bringing up, training, or educating a kid. The parents' and children's ability to maintain a healthy and balanced connection is an important aspect in the development of their bodies and minds. Parents bond with their newborn via physical contact immediately after giving birth, engaging in activities such as holding, carrying, and playing with the infant. The parents are the first teachers of their kid, and they introduce their infant to the world of movement. Parents have the longest, most consistent, and most intimate bond with their kid. A kid's whole family dynamic is based on how they get along with their parents. Attachment between a career and a newborn is the first step in forming a healthy, lifelong parent-child bond. Parenting is taking charge of a child's physical, emotional, and social development and maturation. It also involves the process of giving the kid care and protection. An essential element of successful socialization is the opportunity to develop as a child in a safe and nurturing environment with supportive parents (Vandeleur et. al., 2007). Adolescent children need their parents' unconditional love, care, warmth, and serious attention in order to flourish in their current settings. Adolescent adjustment is heavily influenced by parental involvement. There are two ways of thinking about becoming a parent. In one, the parents are the ones who select how they would act and handle any circumstance involving their kid. On the other side, kids can pick up on their parents' moods and actions no matter what's going on. It's crucial to take into account the way a kid sees his or her parents, since a distorted impression might create irreparable damage to a person's sense of self. It's crucial to attend to kids' wants and needs even at a young age. For the sake of this analysis, "parenting style" refers to how parents are really being regarded by their offspring.

Parenting is a learned skill that gets better with time. A parent is often thought of as sharing a biological connection with their kid. Yet, the act of nourishing, caring for, and protecting may not primarily be biological. Parental parenting philosophies are heavily influenced by culture. Other variables like money, social status, etc. have an influence on parenting style. When their children enter adolescence and experience hormonal changes, parents face a greater struggle. Even now, they are struggling with questions of sexuality and identity. Teenagers often worry that no one, particularly their parents, can relate to their emotions. When it comes to raising a family, everyone wants to know the secret to the perfect parent-child bond. Every parent wants to raise well-behaved, respectful, and responsible children, and they have high hopes for the success of positive parenting practices. Sometimes, parents may educate their kid a wide variety of skills and knowledge without realising it, only to later express regret for doing so. Insight into the current state of the parent-child connection and the issues that are straining it may be gleaned from this study. To be a parent is to take an active role in your child's development on both an emotional and a physical level. The purpose of parenting is to develop children who are successful in all aspects of life, including academics, relationships, and emotions. As a result, parents play crucial responsibilities in directing, supervising, and starting their children's opportunities and social contacts.

A kid learns the most by watching their parents; therefore if they make mistakes in front of their eyes or use inappropriate language, the youngster will pick it up quickly and may even imitate the behaviour or words later on. Yet it's not a simple task to do. It's also crucial to understand that parenting is collaboration between parent and kid, not just a one-way path. When the flowers in a garden all bloom at once, the result is breathtaking. In the same way, if parents develop their "gardening" skills, they will be better able to appreciate their child's unique character and encourage its growth, resulting in a more fruitful and aromatic "garden." All good parents should strive to do this. Background, as the authors call it, has a profound impact on our kids from a young age. Several parent-child interactions have an impact on the child's outcomes and are interconnected. Parenting, which may be thought of as a partnership, entails a wide range of activities that are designed to foster an attachment to the child and prompt predictable patterns of behaviour. It has been argued that families have a sociocultural and economic influence in shaping their children's personalities. Having a parent there at this time of transition from childhood to adulthood is crucial. When parents set limits and rules and engage in meaningful emotional communication with their children, it has a significant influence on the child's emotional growth. Parents may be characterised in a variety of ways, two of which are how responsive they are and how demanding they can be (Fletcher et. al., 2008).

No-Questions-Asked Instruction Parents' primary focus is on setting limits for their children, and their level of control over them is based on how strictly they adhere to those limits. Although if being there for one's children is the most common and defining aspect of parenting, a mother's responsiveness also includes meeting the children's emotional and physical needs. Careful and firm punishment has both been demonstrated to benefit kids' mental health. If a kid's early development takes place in a safe and nurturing environment where his or her requirements for parental involvement are addressed, then that child will have the finest possible foundation upon which to build his or her adult life and engage in the process Adolescents have high expectations of their significant others to satisfy their emotional needs and provide the comfort and love they need from their parents. Parents have a significant role in helping their adolescents develop socially, cognitively, and emotionally.

Many children's development into young adults has been greatly aided by their parents. Caregiving is now recognised as a major factor in a child's later development of interpersonal skills. Feeding, educating, nurturing, and teaching children are all aspects of parenting. To bridge the generation divide, parents need the tools to raise responsible children. Kids don't become spoilt when their parents know how to strike a good balance between enabling and restricting their activities and being too permissive. As a result, they learn how to be effective parents. Separation between parent and child is inevitable when adults lack parenting skills. As their kid enters adolescence, parents need to know how to deal with the changes in their child's behaviour and how it will affect their relationship. Should they fail to do so, they will be in for a rough ride as the youngster develops into adulthood. Parents who are able to maintain acceptable expectations of teenagers are less prone to have erroneous impressions about the complexity of adolescence. In addition, young people of all ages should be reassured that their efforts to grow and improve are worthwhile, and they should not be stifled by criticism or the expectation that they must perform above their capabilities.

Mindful Parenting

Parenting begins long before a kid is born. In fact, it officially starts in the months leading up to conception. As the old adage goes, "once a parent, always a parent," this remains true throughout life. There is a plethora of methods parents use, both overt and covert, to socialise their kids. There could be two sorts of direct effects: hereditary and experiential. Children's genetic composition may be affected by biological factors. Over and beyond this, experience would be a primary stimulant to development, with the experiences offered by parents having a direct impact on their children's growth. And this manifests itself in their thoughts and actions. The goal of mindfulness training is to train one's mind to focus on the now without dwelling on the past or anticipating the future. "It's an intentional practice of being totally present with one's thoughts and emotions," says Pete Loper, a pediatrician and child psychiatrist. Thus, "mindful parenting" refers to the act of incorporating mindfulness into your regular parenting routine. It's the practice of repeatedly choose to focus on the here-and-now with one's own person and one's children. There's a chance that this might make you more open-minded, inquisitive, discriminating, and tolerant. Being introspective and in control of your emotions in their presence is possible.

Mindful Parenting Has Several Elements

- **Self-awareness:** This means being aware of and able to name the emotions triggered by your child's actions.

- **Self-regulation:** The capacity to be with one's emotions rather than act on them in the moment.

- **Empathy:** Being empathetic means being able to recognise and accept your child's emotions, no matter how strong they may be, even if you don't share them. Through empathy, you can affirm your children's feelings and teach them the words to describe them without passing judgement.

- **Intentional hearing:** Listening attentively means taking in your child's words and body language as well.

Mindful parenting may not yet be considered one of the four primary parenting styles, but it is quickly gaining acceptance as a successful method. Mindful parenting differs from other philosophies and approaches because it emphasises being present in the moment rather than prescribing specific actions.

Positive Parenting

The role of a parent is crucial. Bringing up children is an exciting and demanding adventure. Many people, including medical professionals, loved ones, and even total strangers, may offer you guidance as you go. But, every family is different. Positive, healthy connections with children may be fostered via sensitivity and responsiveness on the part of adults. More specific behaviors, such as parental warmth and openness and constant support, constant monitoring and surveillance, a certain degree of autonomy, availability, setting limits and clear rules accompanied by inductive discipline, expectations, and applications depending on the child's age are all components of positive parenting practices. Positive parenting practices include these elements. The healthy development of your child's intellect, self-confidence, capacity to flourish, and even their potential to build connections as they go through life all depend on you showing them love and affection. A healthy early relationship paves the way for kids to grow up and become content, self-sufficient adults. Our capacity to overcome obstacles and bounce back from setbacks is strengthened by loving, stable relationships. These parenting practices are comparable to those of a secure attachment figure and an authoritative style (high levels of responsiveness and high levels of demandingness). Throughout childhood, a kid is more likely to form a secure attachment to a parent if the parent is receptive to the child's needs. The kid will acquire self-assurance in their capacity to engage with the independent world, to confront obstacles, and to control their own emotions as a result of this, which will enable them to safely explore the surrounding environment. Children who have developed strong emotional ties are better able to regulate their own emotions and actions and are more likely to succeed in life. To put it another way, they provide a secure foundation from which the child may go out and study as well as connect with others. "Secure attachment" is the term used by experts to describe this form of close bond between a kid and its caretakers. In spite of hardships like poverty, family instability, parental stress, and despair, children who are securely linked are better equipped to persevere. According to a recent study, roughly six out of every ten kids are able to have emotionally stable relationships with their parents. For the 40% of children who don't have secure attachments, dealing with parental grief may result in avoidance or even resistance. A child obtains the parenting styles that are based on the cultural patterns of the parents. The child's temperament is also a factor. It is the responsibility of parents to ensure their children get a quality education. Youngsters that get sufficient care, freedom and strong management display greater levels of competence. Studies have shown that these kids have developed advanced social skills. Good parenting leads in extra development an ability which includes establishing a strong connection with others, being self-reliant, and independence.

According to the research, this may put youngsters at a far higher risk for developing severe behavioural issues. The government of India uses a variety of commercials, such as those promoting vaccines at the appropriate age, health and cleanliness, the necessity of iron folic acid tablets, universal access to education, and so on, to spread positive parenting concepts and content to the country's parents. Properly nurturing a kid is an investment in our nation's future. Time and circumstance in human civilization have allowed numerous novel ideas and concepts to enter the health and education fields. There have been numerous recent shifts in parenting philosophy that emphasise the significance of parental involvement in their children's growth. Promising programmes to teach parents how to raise children with safe attachments have been piloted by researchers. Children learn to obey rules and control their emotions when their parents are actively involved and provide guidance in these areas. It's crucial to teach youngsters coping mechanisms like creative problem solving as they learn to regulate their emotions and actions. Having these abilities might give people the assurance that they can deal with anything that comes their way. They need to have a conversation about how they feel. Collaborate with them to develop actionable fixes. Remember that when kids become older, meeting their basic need doesn't have to entail catering to their every whim. Always evaluate a child's developmental stage and the skills they need to master at that time. Maybe they are struggling to control their emotions, are unsure of how to act in a certain circumstance, are unsure of how to approach a new job, or are having trouble forming or maintaining friendships. Even if your connection with your kid has become strained and stressful, it is never too late to start working towards a better, more pleasant relationship. Many studies have shown that the bond between parents and their children has a lasting effect on their children's self-esteem, resilience, and overall happiness in adulthood. Parents are the most formative figures in their children's lives. They will have a significant and long-lasting effect. In reality, parents' own upbringing, both good and bad, has a significant impact on the way they raise their own children. Parenting is a dynamic and complicated phenomenon that is shaped by a wide variety of circumstances, including but not limited to, societal norms and expectations, religious views, and the personalities and traits of the children involved.

Being a kind and considerate parent may help put your children up for success, instill in them the ability to exercise self-control, lessen the possibility that they will engage in negative behaviours, and foster an emotionally close bond between you and your children. The best parents know when to use discipline, but they focus on positive reinforcements like attention and praise whenever feasible. Misbehavior consequences work best when:-

- **Reliable And Constant**

To help your kid understand the difference between appropriate and inappropriate behaviour, you may want to consider using consequences. A positive outcome, therefore, is one that a youngster may foreseeable experience if they make a certain decision. When children are provided with clear rules (or given explicit instructions) and the penalties for breaking those rules are implemented consistently, the children might develop a sense of what is right and wrong. Being inconsistent affects the effectiveness of consequences because it makes it more difficult for children to anticipate when they will occur, making it more challenging for them to learn.

- **Implemented Right Away**

The most effective consequences are those that can be experienced right away, since this makes the connection between the behaviour and the result very evident. Younger children may not make the link between their mis-behaviour and its delayed consequences, which may reduce their efficacy. At the age of 2, consequences start to have an effect. When introduced to youngsters any earlier, they lack the requisite cognitive and linguistic development to fully appreciate them (or to make positive choices to avoid them). Younger children have a harder time accepting that there would be long-term repercussions to their actions. So, if a preteen is caught breaking screen time rules on Wednesday, he or she may have less time with technology the following day, Thursday. Modern forms of reinforcement and sanctions, such as behaviour contracts, may be effective with adolescents. It's important to teach your kids responsibility, but avoiding repercussions for too long might get you stuck in a parenting rut.

❖ Logically

Choose a repercussion that seems sense given the circumstances. Your kid should not have a toy to throw, therefore do not give it to him or her. Turn off the TV if your kids are fighting over it. If your kid is being unsafe while playing on the swing, take them off the swing. Children may better understand the relationship between actions and their effects when those outcomes follow logically from one another. In the event that you find yourself unable to come up with a reasonable conclusion, it is helpful to have a few alternative outcomes prepared. Don't use threats of punishment; your kid could start cooperating only when you threaten. Just intervene and execute the punishment gently.

❖ Brief

When our kids make the correct choices, we win as parents. Hence, keep punishments for misbehaviour brief and offer the children another opportunity as quickly as feasible. A small kid won't miss a toy for more than a few minutes. If they continue to make poor decisions after getting a second opportunity, you may extend the duration of the punishment. Try not to think in terms of impractically long periods of time like a full week.

Factors Affecting Parenting

❖ Social Class

The concepts that parents have about parenting and the methods in which they carry out their responsibilities as parents vary significantly depending on a family's financial status. Different socioeconomic groups have different parenting philosophies and approaches. Parents from diverse socioeconomic backgrounds raise their children in different ways, due in part to the vast differences in the environments in which they live and the ways in which they interact with others, including their children. Researchers into childhood are still quite interested in the effects of family socioeconomic status. This curiosity stems from the worry that many children from low-socioeconomic-status families lack access to the same resources and experiences, putting them at risk for developmental problems, and the belief that children from high-socioeconomic-status families afford them a variety of services, goods, parental actions, and social connections that potentially redound to the benefit of children (Bradley and Corwyn,2002). Different parents from various socioeconomic strata bring up their children in different ways, in part as a reaction to the diverse conditions in which they live and in part in response to the different ways in which they interact with the world, including their children. Those who are interested in the development of children continue to find the subject of socioeconomic status to be of significant interest.

This interest stems from the belief that high-socioeconomic-status families provide their children with a variety of services, goods, parental action, and social connections that have the potential to be beneficial to children and from the concern that many children from lower-socioeconomic-status families do not have access to the same resources and experiences, which puts them at risk for developing behavioural and emotional issues (Bradley and Corwyn, 2002). Socioeconomic considerations are a significant contributor to the formation of parenting styles. When it comes to the upbringing of their children, parents from diverse socioeconomic backgrounds often priorities different ideals and work for distinct ends. Lower and working class parents have a tendency to (1) place a greater emphasis on obedience and respect for authority; (2) be more restrictive and authoritarian more frequently using power assertive discipline; (3) reason with their children less frequently; and (4) display less warmth and affection than middle and upper class parents. Why might these contrasting parenting styles exist in the first place? The majority of theories revolve on the pressures that come with living on a low income and how those pressures affect parenting.

Our theory for the relationship between economic circumstances and parenting styles focuses on the abilities that people in various industries require to be able to do their jobs successfully. Because of the nature of their work, some parents from lower socioeconomic classes may, very rationally, place a greater emphasis on deference to authoritative people. Because these are the qualities that are valued in business executives, professionals, and other white collar workers, parents of children from middle and upper class backgrounds are more likely to reason with their children and place a greater emphasis on individual initiative, curiosity, and creativity.

Parents with middle-incomes and those with lower incomes have both developed parenting styles that are well tailored to the specific requirements of the socio-cultural milieu in which they live. When it comes to raising their children, those parents who had children and lived in low-income regions did not use the greatest and most productive parenting techniques. As a consequence, parents in these low-income communities might considerably benefit from additional counseling. One research provided an answer to this issue. It demonstrated how providing parents with the chance to learn about various parenting techniques might be quite beneficial in low-income settings. Implementing parenting programmes that enhanced consistency and positivism in parenting was one answer. Children's ability to engage and manage their emotions was aided by this. Since upper classes were more likely to favour independence rather than compliance, socioeconomic status was also able to predict child engagement. Socioeconomic status influences certain parents' approaches to parenting. Parents from diverse socioeconomic backgrounds typically raise their children differently. An examination of the abilities required by various professions provides one reason for the correlation between economic considerations and parenting methods. It's possible that parents from lower socioeconomic backgrounds stress respect to authority officials since doing so is essential to their livelihood. Since these traits are valued among corporate executives, professionals, and other white collar professions, parents from the middle and upper classes may use this as an argument while raising their children. Parents of all socioeconomic backgrounds have developed approaches to raising children that work effectively within their own cultural contexts.

❖ Gender Of The Child

In Indian culture, male and female children are nurtured differently from a young age. Men are favoured, coddled, and seen as priceless treasures, but females are often regarded as being under men and subject to their authority. Males are given preferential treatment. There is a disparity in the amount of respect and attention given to male and female offspring. Education is one of the most important aspects that might contribute to a shift in mindsets like these. In order to foster national growth and prosperity, it is imperative that both sexes be accorded equal treatment.

❖ Parental Relationships

The children's growth might be negatively impacted when the parents have strained interpersonal relationships. It's possible that some youngsters may blame themselves for the arguments that they get into with their peers, which can have a detrimental effect on their mental and emotional health. Some of the factors that have a negative impact on the interpersonal relationships of the parents and, as a result, the development of their children include things like lack of money, drunkenness, violent relationships in the home, and avoidance.

❖ Parental Education

There is a significant correlation between the amount of education of the parents and the way in which they bring up their children. It is assumed that parents who have completed higher levels of education would provide a more disciplined and capable upbringing for their offspring. Nonetheless, low-income parents who have at least some education often have the expectation that their children would improve in terms of both school and life accomplishments. One study indicated that parents' level of education was positively related to their parenting style. Sixty-five percent of professionals who are also parents want to raise their kids in a more relaxed manner.

What Is Attachment

Infants form attachments with their primary careers because they need to be physically and emotionally close to them in order to feel safe and secure. It's not the case for most other animals; human infants have no innate mobility, nutrition, or defense mechanisms. Babies are hardwired from the start to exhibit behaviours that help them remain in the safe proximity of their primary careers for as long as possible. As parents, we want our children to create solid attachments with us, and that's why we work so hard at encouraging healthy attachment development. The goal may be reached without resorting to extreme tactics. Strike a balance in your life and make the most of the attachment experience by moderation, common sense, and consideration of your personal circumstances. The child's ideal nervous system growth depends on his or her feeling safe, understood, and tranquil. An infant's brain develops in a way that gives him the finest possible start in life: a secure sense of attachment that fosters curiosity, optimism, self-awareness, trust and empathy (Segal et al, 2019). The objective of attachment is not to provide the kid with entertainment or play (the parent's role as a playmate), food (the parent's role as a caretaker), rules (the parent's role as a disciplinarian), or education (the parent's role as a teacher) (this would be the role of the parent as a teacher). Attachment occurs when a youngster views his or her main caregiver as a safe refuge and comforter, as well as a springboard for further exploration. The bond between parents and their children is a crucial emotional connection. Child and parent mental health might be negatively impacted. As a result, parents are more willing to invest in their children because of the closeness they have with them when they have a secure bond to them. Parents that are actively involved in their children's lives are able to spend more time modeling positive conduct for their kids, which in turn helps their kids pick up such habits and stick with them. According to Attachment Theory, children who have secure attachments with their parents are more likely to believe in their own inherent value and to develop healthy self-esteem.

The quality of an adolescent's early attachment relationships with the main careers is essential in predicting the adolescent's academic achievement, according to a review of the relevant research on the topic of attachment and academic performance. To be more specific, there is a connection between having stable attachments and successful results in school. In addition, the study that was looked at shows that responsive and involved parenting is connected with children's cognitive development, their ability to carry out activities, and their resilience. This indicates that those adolescents who had safe attachments as children are more likely to do well in school, at home and conduct well compared to those adolescents who had insecure attachments. Secure attachment, fostered by parental attunement and adequate response, is characterised by a sense of autonomy and mastery over one's surroundings, as well as a trust in and confidence in the reliability and efficacy of others. Children that are securely connected will seek out their carers in times of difficulty, but will also feel comfortable enough to go out on their own during times of relative calm. Instead, insecure anxious-avoidant attachment is linked to parental absence and severe rejection. These kids see the world as harsh and uncaring, and they can't bring themselves to love themselves or others. Children with anxiety avoidance disorder are unwilling to seek comfort from their parents, even in times of difficulty, for fear of being rejected or punished. Attachment anxiety and ambivalence are both linked to parental inconsistency.

Attachment Style

A child's attachment style is the set of behaviours they adopt in order to stay close to their primary career. Four distinct attachment types in children may be identified based on how a newborn responds to his or her primary career throughout infancy and toddlerhood. A child's attachment style is important because the types of attachment styles during childhood continue to have an impact on that individual in adulthood. According to attachment theory (Fisher, 1974), a healthy parent-child bond is crucial to a child's growth and development, while a strained one might put them at greater danger. Parents are protective factors for children to ease behavioral adaption issues, and studies demonstrate that positive parent-child relationships are crucial to their development. The bond that forms between a kid and its primary caretaker is indicative of how that person will come to see the world, themselves, and their connections to others. Attachment styles develop as a consequence of interactions between infants and their primary cares. An internal working model is the set of representations that result from these associations. They have a profound impact on one's sense of self and the world. Children take acquire the traits and behaviours of their role models, including their interpersonal habits and how they cope with stress. Those who have a more optimistic view of the world, for instance, might lean on friends and family to support them through tough times. Those who think the world doesn't care about them, however, will feel abandoned. As a result, people's perceptions will influence their actions and well-being in different ways. There is a mountain of evidence demonstrating the profound importance of parental connection in the formative years of a child's life. The resources to offer not just a safe haven in times of danger but also as a secure platform from which to explore are available to the parent who has developed attachment security and the ability to be a responsive caregiver. Authoritative parenting entails a caring, child-centered approach, yet with defined limits and democratic principles, including providing a safe refuge and stable basis. When kids have a sense of security, love, and care, they flourish. It's not hard for many parents to get connected with their kid. It may be far more challenging for those who did not feel loved, safe, or important when they were little.

Evidence suggests that attachment has a significant impact on both cognitive and social-emotional development in young children. The importance of parental bonding in the formative years of children is supported by a mountain of evidence. Research shows that attachment influences not just cognitive growth but also social and behavioural maturity in young children. Children's attachment experiences are gradually consolidated into what are known as "internal working models" of relationships throughout the course of their lives. The kind and quality of care that parents offer to their offspring may vary greatly (Bowlby, 1973).

How Attachment Style Affects Parenting

The method in which parents interact with their child may be related to how well the child does in school and in social situations. This pattern of attachment describes the special and long-lasting connection that develops between a parent and a kid via their shared experiences and routines in the areas of physical, emotional, and social development. Parent-child connections are thought to have a significant role in shaping children's identities and their outlooks on life. Attachment styles are ways in which people relate to one another. Our upbringing, whether we want to admit it or not, greatly influences our parenting style. Inconsistently maintaining physical closeness to a parent, as well as a desire for personal space and social acceptance, are environmental factors that contribute to the development of anxious attachment. In adults, anxious attachment manifests as a persistent fear of rejection if they are not sufficiently connected to others or recognized for who they are as individuals, leading to significant distress. A parent's attachment type is most strongly predicted by their own attachment style with their own parents, according to studies on attachment. The term "attachment style" is used to describe the mental "working models" we create of how interpersonal bonds operate. Their impact on our relationships with significant others is profound. The security, worry, dread, avoidance, and contentment we experience in our closest connections throughout our lives may be profoundly affected by the bonds we build in our first interactions with cares.

There are numerous negative consequences of developing an insecure attachment style as a youngster. Yet, it is not to say that we must necessarily repeat the mistakes of the past. The good news is that attachment research has also discovered that what predict a person's parenting style are not their childhood experiences but how deeply they have grieved and made meaning of their grief. Even though we had a difficult upbringing, we can change into better people and provide our children with a healthier, more secure connection if we are prepared to investigate and confront the unpleasant aspects of our experience and construct a cohesive narrative out of it. Understanding our attachment type with our parents and other significant cares might help us get insight into our upbringing. It's important to remember that we might experience a wide range of attachment types with other people. As you learn about your attachment type, you may understand into many of your current and former relationships. Among the many elements influencing children' motivation to succeed in school, the parent-child connection has been found to be significant. Parental harshness in terms of punishment, overprotection, and an inability to or unwillingness to deny is all significant predictors of academic pressure. The academic strain of pupils may be significantly reduced or alleviated when parents and children have a strong connection. Peer pressure becomes more pervasive as youngsters get integrated into school communities. Research shows that middle and upper primary school pupils have stronger relationships with their peers than they do with their parents. The term "peer relationship" may mean a variety of things, but most often it refers to the kind of interpersonal connection that is formed and nurtured via conversation between people who are the same age or who have comparable levels of psychological development.

- **Secure Attachment-** A baby that is firmly bonded has parents who are actively engaged in their life. It's the perfect combination of security, love, freedom, and adventure. A baby, who is firmly bonded, for instance, may play with an engaging toy but eventually crawl back to her mother for comfort. A parent who is comfortable both expressing their affection and letting their kid explore the world around them is more likely to foster a secure bond. A kid who has stable attachments develops a sense of confidence in others and in the world around them, learning that those closest to them can be relied upon to offer them with space when needed while still providing them with closeness and nurturing.

A child that has formed a stable connection to their career views that person as a safe haven from which they may explore the world. They know they have the freedom to explore on their own, but that they can always return to the parent's protection. Securely connected children develop a "working model" of relationships based on the belief that their loved ones will always be there for them. Youngsters who are able to build solid attachments are better able to keep their individuality as adults while still having meaningful relationships. They may have confidence in which they are and practice positive interpersonal skills. My blog post, "How Your Attachment Style Changes Your Relationship," goes into further detail regarding how people's childhood attachment patterns may shape their adult relationships. Parents who can provide an emotionally safe atmosphere and control their own responses will help their children bond securely. The parents might also have a role in their child's development in this area. Parents that are able to foster a solid bond recognise their child's uniqueness and respond sensitively to his or her needs. They understand the child's feelings and may just "be there" for them. Nonetheless, this does not imply that parents should be without flaws. Nobody pays constant attention to their child.

- **Preoccupied Attachment-** For children, having a parent who is only sometimes present might lead to an anxious or preoccupied attachment style. The kid of such parents often feels confused and upset because of the parent's erratic availability and rewards. Preoccupied attachment parents were unable to provide love and comfort. They loved when convenient. They might be cold, aloof, or abusive. Children with narcissistic or borderline parents frequently have preoccupied attachment. Preoccupied attachment kids learn to be hyper vigilant around their parents, attempting to be there for love moments while guarding against being injured.

- Preoccupied adults are envious and clingy. They're clingy and distrustful in partnerships. They're making up for their parents' inconsistent affection. In maturity, they want to manage their spouse and be there. As you may guess, this typically pushes couples away, making the preoccupied partner more nervous. The needs of the parent are often put on the back burner as the parent looks to the child for fulfillment. When children show "emotional hunger," it drains them emotionally and provides a poor replacement for genuine care and affection. If a parent isn't addressing a kid's emotional needs, the youngster may become overly attached to that parent or exhibit worrisome behaviour while around that parent. When a kid develops this attachment style, they internalise the "working model" that they must be hyper vigilant and attentive in all of their interactions in order to have their needs satisfied. Anxious attachment style occurs when a youngster has trouble believing that others will be there for them in times of need.

Yet even as adults, they may struggle with feelings of neediness or insecurity in close friendships and partnerships. This is why it is as crucial for us as parents to never seek validation or affection from our children. It is crucial for the benefit of our kids that we satisfy our own adult needs via relationships with other adults. It's crucial to take stock of how frequently we rely on our kids to boost our own self-esteem. When it comes to our interactions with and responses to our children, we also need to be mindful of how often we are preoccupied or inconsistent.

- **Avoidant Attachment-** Although the parent with an avoidant attachment may provide for the kid's material requirements, they may struggle to connect with the child emotionally. A parent might seem like an "emotional desert" to a kid. Children in such homes learn that pretending they have no wants is the surest way to get their needs satisfied by their parents. They adjust by distancing themselves from their feelings and adopting a sham "independent" position. For a youngster with this attachment style, the "functioning model" of relationships teaches them to keep their needs and wishes to themselves and to maintain an emotional distance from others. Children who don't develop intimate emotional bonds with their careers early in life may struggle to identify and act on their own wants as adults, or to take emotional risks in romantic relationships.

  As they reach adults, they may have trouble forming close relationships because they have a hard time exhibiting emotion or needing help from others. They reject their spouses' efforts at intimacy because they see it as "needy." They may have trouble recalling specifics from their youth and may believe that their formative years had no bearing on who they were as adults. There has to be an emotional connection and availability between ourselves and our kids. Just providing for a child's necessities is not enough. Understanding our own tendencies towards introspection and emotional detachment is crucial.

- **Disorganized Attachment**- When a parent either causes or experiences fear from their kid, an insecure connection develops. The parent's response in this case is unpredictable. A parent may laugh and praise one conduct one minute and then lash out angrily at the same behaviour the next. Children lack a systematic approach to getting their needs satisfied as a result of their irregular and unpredictable behaviour. They're terrified and there's nothing they can do. But, the closer they get near their parent, the more terrified they get. If you want your child to feel safe and comfortable, you need to be consistent. As a substitute, kids are receiving a parent who may be downright scary. Without a sense of fundamental protection, these youngsters typically demonstrate emotional upheaval and a bewildering combination of behaviours. Anxiety and avoidance in romantic partnerships are common reactions to this attachment pattern in adults. If they are feeling desperate or needy when someone pushes away, they may be distant and withdrawn while someone is trying to reconnect with them. While in a relationship, they often act in ways that are both unpredictable and frightening to their partner.

To know who we are as individuals and as parents, it helps to know how our experiences as children shaped who we are now. We may learn a lot about how we could act as a parent by reflecting on the impact our early attachments had on the way we learnt to interact. But, regardless of our attachment type, excellent parenting always begins with looking within and facing the inevitable grief we suffered as children. A strong, secure connection with us as parents is possible if we focus on ourselves and create more positive "working models" of relationships. But, we must be honest and centre our attention on ourselves if we want that to occur. Self-compassion is crucial when we investigate our attachment history and its potential effects on our current relationships. If we want to alter our attachment pattern, we'll have to put in time and effort to processing our deepest childhood wounds. Emotions may arise throughout this process, but we must remember to stay on our own sides. Developing an awareness of who you are is a crucial aspect of maturing into a fully realised person.

Attachment And Parenting

Attachment is a fundamental human need that, when satisfied, results in the development of close personal relationships. In this process, the child's parents are the child's first instructors, and it is highly crucial for the child's development of social adaption that they be given this role. According to the Bioecological Systems theory, the maturation of children's adaptive capabilities is shaped by the interaction of their features with the proximal processes and the environment that they are exposed to throughout time. Attachment between a parent and a kid is a very significant proximal process in human development, and it will continue to have an effect on the psychological and behavioral development of children. The term "attachment" refers to a kind of profound, long-lasting, personal, and secure emotional connection that develops as a result of contact between an individual and their parents. This connection is known as the parent-child attachment. A primary objective of attachment parenting is the development of a secure connection between parent and child. Those that practice this approach to parenting make an effort to be responsive to their child's needs in a timely manner, as well as emotionally accessible to them around the clock. Some people think that if a kid has a solid relationship to one or both of its parents, they will grow up to be more confident, empathetic, and at ease. Those who support attachment parenting are often anti-vaccination activists who advocate for natural births, a family bed, no spanking, and home schooling. A child's upbringing is one of the most important factors in determining whether or not they will acquire the capacity for empathy. When a kid's parents treat them with hostility or when the youngster experiences a great deal of rejection from his or her parents, the child develops the mindset that this behaviour is typical and that this is the way that life should be lived. As a result, as this youngster grows up, he turns his back on the people around him, certain that it is perfectly OK to behave in this manner and that this is how everyone else acts. But what he does not realise is that the people around him, who have probably had good parenting and upbringing and have a good emotional understanding, are seeking emotional support from him but are not receiving it, and as a result, are getting hurt. He does not realise this because he does not realise that the people around him have likely had good parenting and upbringing and have a good emotional understanding. Because of this, his interactions with other people are difficult to maintain. To a lesser extent than intrusiveness, detachment, and psychological issues on the part of the parents themselves (Speranza et al., 2020), attachment style is a major determinant in shaping parenting practises. Providing care is a byproduct of a more complex behavioural system, the attachment system, which develops in tandem with the need for care (George and Solomon, 1999). When mothers fear for the safety of their children, the fundamental goal of the care giving system is to provide opportunities for physical closeness and reassurance. Maternal sensitivity, or the capacity to recognise and react correctly to a child's emotions, is a key factor in mothers' success in maintaining their offspring's sense of safety. Individuals' functioning, especially in the formation of meaningful relationships, is influenced by the internal working models, which tend to be rather constant over the lifetime. Adult attachment has been shown to be significant in a variety of ways, including parenting style, romantic relationships, and psychological and physiological well-being. The introduction of self-report questionnaires that have been shown to accurately evaluate normal thoughts, emotions and actions in the setting of intimate relationships has contributed to the explosion of research on adult attachment. When parents and children have strained relationships, children lose the trust and emotional grounding essential for effective communication, and they develop a deficit in the knowledge and abilities necessary for healthy social interaction. Numerous research have indicated that teenagers' negative emotions, subjective well-being, loneliness, depression, and risk-taking behaviors are influenced by their peers, which is consistent with the indirect impact model of the parent-child influence mechanism (Zhang et al., 2019).

Confidence in others' emotional availability to give reassurance in times of pain and/or need is the definition of attachment security. In contrast, the heightened demand for intimate relationships that characterises attachment anxiety stems from a person's belief that they lack the resources to deal with stress and danger on their own. Anxious-attached people employ these hyperactive techniques to get their significant others (who they believe aren't being protective or supportive enough) to pay more attention to them (Shaver and Mikulincer, 2002). Discomfort with proximity and a focus on emotional distance and autonomy manifest themselves in the form of repressed support seeking, which is a hallmark of attachment avoidance. These deactivation methods are used by avoidant people so that they don't have to feel the distress that results from the absence of their attachment figures. To investigate the link between parental attachment and parenting quality, a number of researches have used self-report questionnaires (Jones et al., 2015). Attachment insecurity has been linked to high levels of stress and arousal in parent-infant interactions, whereas secure attachment has been linked to resilience in the face of adversity and a more flexible approach to parenting. Li et al. (2021) discovered that whereas maternal anxiety was adversely associated with the quality of the connection between mothers and their adolescents, maternal avoidance was similarly associated with the quality of the relationship between dads and their adolescents. The quality of these mothers' relationships with their adolescents was predicted by their levels of attachment anxiety, but not by their levels of avoidance.

Attachment Theory And Eating Disorders

A parent's capacity to care for and nurture a kid may be negatively impacted by the parent's own eating disorder, which may manifest itself in an unhealthy concern with one's own body, a fear of becoming overweight, and a disordered approach to food preparation and consumption. Abnormalities in the way people form attachments have been connected to eating disorders (Illing et al., 2010).Eating disorders are problems of mental health in which a person attempts to use food as a form of coping with difficult emotions and circumstances in their lives. This presents itself as various habits around food, such as eating excessively or insufficiently, as well as being preoccupied with one's body weight and form. An established risk factor for the development of an eating problem is a pattern of attachment that is characterized by feelings of insecurity. Studies have revealed that between 70 to 100 percent of patients who suffer from anorexia nervosa also has an insecure attachment style. This may seem like a generalization, but the findings of this research back it up. These findings also demonstrate that those with insecure attachment patterns are more likely to suffer from various types of eating disorders. In addition, this finding was not restricted to those who had been diagnosed with a particular eating problem. An insecure connection was revealed to be a risk factor for disordered eating behaviors, which do not quite meet the criteria for a diagnosis of an eating disorder. Patterns like these include chronic overeating, obsessive eating, and an increased concern on appearance. There is evidence to show that insecure attachment is a risk factor for the indications of an eating disorder before the condition actually reveals itself. Concerns about being overweight, being unhappy with one's body shape, trying to control one's eating or engaging in binge eating are some examples of these warning signals. Excessive or inadequate eating, as well as preoccupation with one's physique, is symptoms of this disorder. Hence, it's fair to say that insecure attachment patterns are frequently the root cause of the psychological and emotional problems that manifest as eating disorder symptoms.

There is evidence to suggest that women who are experiencing symptoms of an eating problem may exercise more discipline in their interactions with their children at mealtime. The mothers with eating disorders have been observed to disengage from the feeding scenario. Researchers have looked at how moms with eating disorder symptoms feed their children, but they have paid less attention to how people with eating disorders parent in general. Evidence from the past suggests that authoritative parenting is related with better results for children than either authoritarian or permissive styles. Of course, not everyone who has trouble with their attachments is also struggling with their weight. Moreover, not all people who struggle with an eating problem also have attachment issues. Some persons developing an eating problem may not necessarily have an insecure attachment type. Eating disorders are influenced by a number of factors, including inability to control emotions, excessive striving for perfection, poor self-esteem, and inappropriate coping techniques. Many of these issues are linked to a lack of trust in relationships. In addition, these elements all have a role in keeping the symptoms of eating disorders alive and well. All adult women with eating problems were shown to be nervously attached in a research. This research also found that these women had little unresolved feelings of trauma or loss, particularly in relation to their moms. This result is consistent with the conclusions of previous research that explore the impact that a mother's own unresolved trauma might have on her capacity to react compassionately to her child's needs. As a consequence, it's possible that trauma might be passed down from generation to generation, playing a pivotal influence in how severe an eating problem becomes. So, taking into account not just the pain experienced by the adolescent, but also by the mother, may help us get a more nuanced understanding of the origins of eating disorders. It's an interesting observation that children of worried moms may struggle to find their own identity since their mothers force their own wants on them. Most study results are based on self-reports from persons who suffer from eating disorders, and as a result, dads are generally overlooked. Yet, the few studies that have looked at the father's part in the onset of an eating disorder have revealed that an insecure attachment to a father figure might make one more vulnerable to developing an eating disorder. When a father figure is absent or distant, dominating, and uninvolved, their kid is more likely to restrict their food intake, worry about their weight, and care about how they look. Surely, additional research on the father's influence in the development of eating disorders would definitely reveal some fascinating discoveries. Attachment qualities may also alter with age (Pinquart et al., 2013); hence, the age difference between the groups may potentially contribute to the variations that were discovered between the people who suffer from eating disorders. There is a high rate of co-occurrence between eating disorders and mood disorders. In general, greater levels of depression are seen in most eating pathologies, and there is a high rate of co-occurrence between eating and mood disorders. One way to think about the function of attachment in patients who suffer from eating disorders is as a system that acts as a mediator between the patients' own experiences and the behaviors of others that help to keep the symptoms alive.

Parent Child Relationship

Because of how influential mothers and fathers are in shaping their children's personalities, values, attitudes, temperaments, coping mechanisms, and overall physical and cognitive growth, parent-child relationships are of paramount significance. The relationship between a parent and a kid is one that helps the child grow in all aspects of their being, including their body, their emotions, and their relationships with other people. It is a special connection that may be enjoyed and fostered by each and every kid and parent. This bond forms the basis for the child's personality, the decisions they will make throughout their life, and their general behaviour. In addition to this, it may have an impact on their level of social, physical, mental, and emotional well-being. As metropolitan lives have drawn a distinct line between at-home care and a child's official education, parenting has been a hot issue of controversy in recent years. Parental authoritarianism is characterised by a lack of response and a high level of expectation. Parents that choose this approach place a greater premium on obedience and compliance, and their children learn to respect authority with less affection and explanation. In addition, authoritarian parents are not very involved with or trust their children. They tend to restrict a child's freedom of expression and enforce rigid rules on his or her behaviour. In other words, the stereotype of authoritarian parents is that they are harsh and demanding, with the view that their children should always act morally and responsibly. Authoritarian parents prioritise maintaining order in the home at the expense of their children's independence and closeness to them. It may be stated that authoritarian parenting relies on regulations that are seen to be tangible since the primary focus of this parenting style is on the conventional family structure and the kid is expected to obey the parent's directions without question.

Individual growth, according to developmental situation theories, is a byproduct of the combined effects of one's home and formal education environments. School, together with the home, plays a significant role in the development of children and teenagers. Thus, we investigated a significant emotional element, scilicet; school bonding that has been frequently linked to adaptability. The fact that parents of multiple children have to divide their attention and resources inequitably based on gender and the number of children in the family helps to explain why only children have a stronger sense of attachment to their parents than those who have siblings. A child's education at home and in a formal setting must be distinct because of the differences between the teacher-student connection and the parent-child relationship. Parents have an obligation to provide a safe and stimulating environment where their children may flourish. This refers to more than just a person's material well-being; it also emphasises their spiritual, intellectual, emotional, and physical progress. Parents have the primary duty of providing their children with the necessities of life, including a safe and stable home, enough clothes, and nutritious food. Parents also have a responsibility to prevent anything that can harm their child's mind from interfering with his or her ability to learn and grow. The term "intellectual security" describes a setting that is conducive to a child's physical and mental growth. To educate a kid is to provide him or her access to a setting that may shape not just his or her cognitive abilities but also his or her moral and ethical foundations. Parenting entails actions, yet those actions cannot happen without a kid. Thus, it's safe to assume that parenting is impossible if there aren't any kids around. A parent's parenting style may be thought of as an umbrella term including their worldview, parenting objectives, and daily habits (Kumar and Fernandez 2017). Understanding the connection between parent-child attachment, school bonding, and social adaption is crucial since it is a well recognized indication of mental health. Several psychological effects have been linked to the quality of the parent-child connection, either directly or indirectly, according to a number of researches (Stefan and Avram, 2017). Moreover, the parent-child attachment provides the foundation for the growth of school bonding, according to both the developmental systems theory and the individual developmental context theory.

Factors Affecting Parent-Child Relationship

- **Social Problems**- Isolation, loneliness, lack of confidence, school troubles, learning issues, anxiety and depression, alcohol and drug misuse (especially connected with mental illness), suicide or self-harming, theft and criminal behaviour are some of the symptoms that may be associated with mental illness.

- **Educational Problems**- factors such as lower learning abilities and academic accomplishments, disruptive behaviour, and bullying.

- **Issues With Discipline**- behaviours such as narcissism, disobedience, instability, recklessness, dishonesty, violence, and disruption in the workplace are all examples of unacceptable conduct.

- **Parental Factors**- Conflict and strife in the family may be caused by a lack of structure and discipline, disagreements on childrearing, and other factors. A level of parental control that is excessive, Anxiety in childhood, being overprotected as a youngster, Marriage discord, divorce or separation, partum depression.

- **Psychosis**- Compared to households without stepchildren, reconstituted families are more likely to have mental problems. Moreover, mental illnesses were more prevalent in households with no employed parents, families with at least one member receiving a disability benefit, and families with lower levels of educational achievement.

- **Eco-Factors**- Compared to families with a parent in a higher professional group, those with low gross weekly incomes and those whose parent worked in a regular occupation had a greater prevalence of mental problems. Also, compared to those who owned their homes, they were more prevalent among people who lived in the social sector.

Suggestive Measures For Parents

The inability of a parent and kid to comprehend one another is a typical source of tension in the relationship between a parent and their child. This tension may be stressful for everyone involved. While there will always be some level of stress in each person's life, the purpose of this article is to make an attempt to reduce the amount of tension that exists between a parent and a kid in order to foster a positive and healthy atmosphere inside the home.

- **Communication-** If there is communication between parents and children from the start, the connection between them will improve. When parents and children are able to talk things out and figure out what each person is expecting, everyone wins.

- **Dynamic**- A parent-child bond evolves with time, much as the human intellect and heart. The connection between parents and children is like a roller coaster since it is always changing, which may be exciting at times but is usually rather terrifying. As a result, it's important for parents to remember this and exercise patience.

- **Consistency**- If a parent makes an effort and can see things from their child's perspective; the two of them will have a more positive connection. The parent may accomplish this by partaking in the same activities as their children, such as reading the same books, seeing the same movies, having the same celebrity crush, playing the same card and board games, eating at the same restaurants, and binge-watching the same television shows. The parent may learn more about the child's likes and dislikes this way. It will also offer those more in common to talk about, strengthening their friendship in the process. As a bonus, this will help the parent better comprehend their youngster.

- **Mealtime**- Having everyone in the family eat together and know where everyone else is at all times is important for maintaining a healthy parent-child connection. It is recommended to start conversations on the day's highlights and low points.

- **Involvement in Academics and Extracurriculars**- The child craves approval, so when he does well on an exam or wins a game, he expects his parents to be ecstatic for him. A parent has a responsibility to pick up and drop off their child to school, lessons, and activities, as well as to attend parent-teacher conferences and games whenever possible. The parent should take advantage of this opportunity to become the first person the kid feels comfortable telling everything about his day at school and on the football field to, in a manner, demonstrate good listening so the youngster knows he is properly listened to.

- **Playfully**- For better relations with their child, parents should occasionally joke around and pull their child's leg. In doing so, the child will learn that he or she can do the same and share stories about what he or she does at that age, and the parents, if appropriate, can do the same by sharing stories from their own childhoods. The kid prefers staying at home and taking car rides with his or her parents when things are relatively calm outside.

- **Openly**- The youngster thrives in environments where there is honest dialogue and unconditional love. When parents are also unafraid to broach taboo subjects like infidelity, drug use, and smoking with their children, the family dynamic improves. When these kinds of conversations arise, parents should ensure their children fully comprehend all sides of any issue. A youngster who often hears both parents' perspectives is less likely to make poor decisions.

- **Workplace Stress** - Parents should separate work and home. Office stress might cause unneeded confrontations and a stressful home. When parents bring work tension home, their conduct changes, and the kid finds it hard to convey significant and tiny things since they know the answer won't be good. Be cool and keep your youngster stress-free.

- **Disagreement**- It's important for parents and children to see disagreements as opportunities for growth. It's possible to make a good choice after some healthy debate and mutual knowledge of the issues at hand. The parent-child bond develops as a result of all these little things. Although raising children is no easy task, being a good parent is not impossible if you put in the time and effort.

Concept Of Parenting Styles

Diana Baumrind, a developmental psychologist at the University of California, Berkeley, is widely credited for influencing the parenting approaches now used in the field of psychology. Baumrind made this observation in the 1960s and found that pre-scholars' behaviour varied widely. There was a strong connection between parenting styles and each kind of behaviour. According to Baumrind, the way in which parents raise their kids has a significant impact on how that kid turns out as an adult. Parenting styles have both direct and indirect effects on children's social development within the context of family life. For example, parents can help their children develop socially competent behaviour patterns by providing opportunities for them to interact with and learn from their peers at home and in the community (Smart & Sanson, 2003). When kids reported feeling their parents had too much power over them, they were more likely to report feeling sad. The use of an authoritative parenting style has been proven to be associated with high levels of psychological health. The perspectives of the parents are a significant factor in influencing the perspectives and behaviours that will be shown by the kid. In the context of child rearing, the term "parenting" refers to the privilege or obligation that falls on the mother and the father, either jointly or separately, to educate the kid in regards to society and culture.

Diana Baumrind, a developmental psychologist, is often credited as the first scientist to study parental approaches (Joshi, Sharama and Mehra, 2009). Every parent acknowledges that raising children is one of the most difficult jobs in the world. Family life and the manner in which parents raise their children are two of the most influential factors in a child's overall social and scholastic development. In addition, parenting is the foundation of a family environment because, in the absence of parental education, it is impossible for parents to successfully execute the tasks and responsibilities that they have been assigned within the family and the larger community. "behaviours and techniques employed by parents to govern and socialise children" are what are meant by the phrase "parenting style" (Lightfoot, Cole & Cole,2009) The connection between parents and their children plays a crucial part in the process of teenage socialisation because it helps to moderate and mediate the effect of influences both inside and outside the home. The connection that a teenager has with his or her parents is, and will continue to be, the one that has the biggest impact. Parental behaviour developed as a complement to the physiological mechanics of reproduction during the course of evolution. In other words, it is believed that parental behaviour developed during a time when fertilised eggs did not mature, hatch, and lead to the survival of the offspring. The approaches to childrearing or the behaviours of parents may be analysed in terms of a wide variety of various qualities, such as acceptance, affection, control, warmth, permissiveness, restrictiveness, and demandingness. In addition to serving as a barometer for offering feedback between parent and newborn, research suggests that varied parenting approaches (including establishing limits and regulations) affect children's mental wellbeing. Previous studies documented the significant links between tough parenting, parental punishment, and teenage problems.

Every parent has their own unique set of routines, beliefs, and expectations for their newborn and these are reflected in how they treat their kid. Family characteristics, such as parents' level of education, parental expectations, parental support, etc., seem to have some effect on teenagers' success drive. Studies have uncovered a wide range of characteristics that play significant roles in forecasting the drive of teenagers to succeed. The term "parenting style" refers to a psychological concept that includes common techniques used by parents. As children grow and mature their parents' approaches to childrearing change to reflect the nuances of their developing personalities. Adolescence is a transitional time when teenagers seek and crave independence, and the stage of infancy is marked by parents' adjustment and adaptation to a new way of life in terms of connecting with their problems. It is crucial to make a distinction between parenting styles and parenting techniques. Parenting techniques are "particular behaviours that parents employ to socialise their children," as Darling and Steinberg put it in 1993, while parenting style is "the emotional milieu in which parents raise their children," as Christopher Spera (2005) writes in his overview of the relevant research. 'Parenting style is characterised as a constellation of attitudes towards the kid that are transmitted to the child and that, taken together, produce an emotional atmosphere in which the parents' behaviours are exhibited' (Darling & Steinberg 1993). The goal of good parenting is to help children adapt to the norms of their community. Yet, there are generalisations that can be made about what makes for excellent parenting. By studying what kinds of parenting best prepare children for life in modern society, we may make great strides in improving the lives of all children. A parenting style is an individual's approach to childrearing (Okoli. et. al 2020).

Psychologists have classified a variety of parenting styles. Authoritative, authoritarian, permissive and uninvolved parents are the four types of parenting styles identified by Baumrind (1991).

a) **Authoritative: -** Like an authoritative father, this style aims to keep the youngster in check, but does so by objectively fair and issue-based encouragement. According to popular belief, the most typical approach to raising children is letting them do anything they want and punishing them according to a set of predetermined standards of behaviour. They give their kids a tone of praise and praise for work, but they expect a lot from them. Help your adolescent take ownership of their life without letting them completely go amok. Parents are characterised and evaluated based on their interactions with their offspring, but kids ultimately look to their parents for guidance. Research shows that adolescents raised by authoritative figures are better able to negotiate differences and take part in debates in which their opinions will be taken seriously. As a result, individuals would have a broader perspective on the world and improved capacity for making choices based on their own values. Most authoritative parents have other goals than just ensuring their children obey the rules. The independence a youngster develops is valued and fostered. They hope their children will learn to be responsible and mature adults who respect themselves and others. And they go about achieving these goals by providing both practical guidance and moral backing. Researchers have characterised authoritative parents as being very demanding (like authoritarian parents) but also highly receptive to their children's needs (Maccoby and Martin 1983).

b) **Authoritarian:-** Parental authoritarianism is characterised by a harsh tone and a heavy hand in disciplining their children. They are strict disciplinarians who want their child to follow their every order, no matter how unpleasant. It's not appropriate for authoritative parents to speak to their adolescent directly, and they shouldn't bring up rules and expectations for the family. Authoritarian parents want their children to blindly comply with their rules and routines. Teens whose parents are overbearing often value obedience to the rules and close monitoring more than independence. In turn, adolescents may become rebellious or too reliant. This refers to a style of parenting where rules and discipline are strictly enforced. They are quite controlling, and they don't let their kids be themselves. Children with authoritarian parents are often restricted in their actions and choices. Instead of using rules and consequences, they use incentives and punishments. The victim is often subjected to physical abuse and is met with emotional distance. In addition, they are overbearing parents that make choices without consulting their offspring. They solely utilise control, despite there being far better methods to develop children to be responsible adults. It's fair to say that authoritarian parents are just like authoritative ones, but with a lot more rules and regulations.

A lack of parental warmth, aggression, and emotional reactivity are common characteristics of these parents. It also involves strict punishments and disciplinary methods, as well as extensive monitoring of the child's day-to-day activities and strong mental stimulation at home. Parents who aren't actively engaged in their children's lives could try to force their children to succeed by replacing free time with extracurricular activities like courses or tutoring. In order to keep the peace and inculcate excellent values in their children, authoritarian parents are convinced that they must exert strict authority over their offspring. There is a lot of physical abuse, strict rules, and coldness involved. A child's parents often want him or her to follow their instructions without inquiry or complaint. When it comes to their children, authoritarian parents have one primary objective: to make their children act in accordance with their standards, regardless of the children's input or preferences. When parents exercise excessive authority over their children, the children lose whatever feeling of individuality they may have had. It sends the message that the child's perspective doesn't matter, which might have negative effects on their growth and development. The children of authoritative parents are less likely to suffer from anxiety, poor self-esteem, and other personality and mental health issues. The assumption that authoritarian parenting is effective because it produces compliant, respectful children is erroneous. Yet as adults, they struggle with low self-esteem, hostility towards their parents, and other personality or mental health disorders.

c) **Permissive:** - Warm and welcoming, permissive parenting is effective. Instead of being actively engaged, they are either indulgent or uncaring; rather than progressively offering autonomy, they let kids make a lot of choices for themselves while they are still capable of doing so. Permissive parents are hospitable, but they have strict rules about what their children should and should not do. Baumrind asserts that "permissive" parents are those that pay attention to their children yet aren't too strict. Children may lack the ability to establish boundaries for themselves if they are not expected to behave maturely. Children may benefit from this by learning to rely on themselves and develop their own interests and skills. There is a risk that it will lead to a lack of self-control. Being a friend to their kid comes before being a parent in the eyes of permissive parents. Those that practice permissive parenting tend to be warm and open with their kids, treating them more like friends than children. Many of them give in too much to their teens and are too passive; thinking that giving them what they want is the best way to show their love for them. Parents who never say "no" to their kids also never disappoint them. Teens are allowed to make many decisions independently of their parents, which is good for their maturation. In most cases, adults shouldn't perceive themselves as major factors in shaping the choices of teenagers, but rather as guides, as if the young actively seek out their counsel. Further research is required, but it seems that teenagers raised by liberal parents don't learn much about boundaries or rule-following, especially if they are less confident in themselves. This broadens Adolescents' interactions with their peers are often motivated by a desire for power and fame, making it difficult for them to exhibit self-control. People generally agree that the results of a permissive upbringing are preferable to those of an authoritarian one but less so than those of an authoritative one. Strong intercommunication and self-control measures are the foundation for the permissive parenting style. Rather of doing it for them, parents are letting their children take charge of their appearance in this trend. They do not place excessive expectations on the children or punish them severely for even slight infractions. Parents provide their children love and care, and in exchange they want their children to act responsibly and maturely. The degree of responsibility is higher than the amount of effort required. Parents who are more permissive encourage their children to self-regulate. Permissive parenting is characterized by an increased emphasis on dialogue and a more relaxed attitude toward discipline. Without clear boundaries in place, children raised with a lax approach are more likely to get into trouble. No parent can expect their kid to perform appropriately in response to being given more independence.

d) **Uninvolved:** - The characteristics of an uninvolved parenting style include that there are minimal expectations placed on the child, a low level of response, and very little communication. Lackadaisical parents like to offer their kids a lot of independence and seldom get in their way. Some parents may deliberately choose this approach, while others may be disinterested in or uncertain of how to raise their children. None of the standard methods of discipline are used. A parent who isn't actively engaged in their kid's life is often too uninformed or unconcerned about the child's welfare to prevent the youngster from doing largely what he wants. It's hard to get a message through. The parents in this group aren't exactly warm and fuzzy. Children are not expected to do much of anything. Many parenting philosophies may be recognised by their distinctive characteristics and their corresponding approaches to child rearing. They provide for the child's necessities, but they aren't involved in the child's life beyond that. They may make sure their kids are fed and given a place to sleep, but that's about all they do in terms of parenting.

There's a chance these parents come out as uncaring, inattentive, and dismissive. There are occasions when such parents ignore or disdain their children. It's also possible that they're abusive in other ways, such as physically or psychologically. Note that free-range parenting is not the same as uninvolved parenting. Free-range parents, in contrast to uninvolved ones, take an active interest in their children's life while yet allowing them significant independence. One should not assume that a parent is not interested in their child's life just because they are too busy with work or other commitments. Intention and concern are crucial. Parents who spend what little spare time they have with their children and make arrangements for their care when they can't be there because of work are not absent. Researchers in the field of developmental psychology have long been curious in the impact that different parenting methods have on the maturation of children. Finding true cause-and-effect links between certain tactics used by parents and the eventual conduct of children is a very challenging endeavour. For instance, it is possible for children who are brought up in very different surroundings to subsequently have personalities that are surprisingly similar to one another. On the other hand, children who are raised in the same setting might have quite distinct personalities while sharing the same upbringing. The rules and love and affection of the negligent parent are often low. They don't disturb kids unless there's an emergency, and they generally leave them alone. Adolescents of uninvolved parents tend to engage in more externalizing behavior because they do not have the structure or control over their lives that adolescents of engaged parents have. Adults with this disorder often struggle with poor self-esteem, immaturity, and familial alienation, and they may exhibit truancy and delinquency habits as children. For instance, a lack of parental involvement has been linked to a variety of antisocial behaviors in children, from vandalism and small theft to assault and rape, according to the study's authors.

These parents tend to offer assurances but fail to follow through. This is a major failing on their side as parents because it causes their children to mistrust them. These may be much more harmful to children when combined with the characteristics of the dominant parent. The well-rounded parent is the one who is in command of the situation, has set boundaries, and communicated them to their offspring. A good parent respects and values their children, shows them affection, and at the same time sets high standards for proper conduct. They don't compromise discipline for affection or vice versa, but rather see kids as whole people with their own preferences and treat them as such. Experts in child psychology believe that a parent's, and especially a father's, ability to empathise with and understand his young kid is a crucial factor in shaping the child's developing personality. Recent research in psychology and education has placed a strong emphasis on the intricacy of the relationship between parents and their children and their academic achievement among different non-cognitive aspects or determinants. Nurturing and supporting children while they are young is one of the most important things a parent can do for their development. The more secure parents are, the more socially adept their children will be (self esteem, moral behaviour, academic achievement and vocational achievement). One has to be patient, persistent, keep in contact, and love to provide support for another person. The parenting style of a family may have a significant impact on a child's development in many different domains, including their social and intellectual competence.

A child whose parents aren't actively involved in their lives is less likely to succeed in almost every field. Deficits in learning, bonding, emotional regulation, and social interactions are common among children with autism. Uninvolved parents are more likely to have been brought up in the same manner. They may find themselves perpetuating the same behaviors and beliefs they were taught to hold true even as adults. It's possible that parents who adopt this strategy do so because they're too preoccupied with their own life to provide much attention to their kids. The parenting style of a family may have a significant impact on a child's development in many different domains, including their social and intellectual competence. The outcomes for children with uninvolved parents are dismal across the board. Deficits in learning, bonding, emotional regulation, and social interactions are common among children with autism. Uninvolved parents are more likely to have been brought up in the same manner. They may find themselves perpetuating the same behaviors and beliefs they were taught to hold true even as adults. It's possible that parents who adopt this strategy do so because they're too preoccupied with their own life to provide much attention to their kids.

The research suggests that the traits, attitudes, and abilities necessary for a successful profession are mostly inherited from one's parents. These traits and attitudes include the capacity to make choices, get along with people, and speak one's mind. In past literature, analyses of various parenting styles have relied heavily on the notion of parental authority. "Low parental control" refers to a situation in which parents are not too involved in their children's daily activities, while "disengagement" describes a situation in which there are no rules or regulations in place and no instruction given. Freedom without a lack of either tight norms or complete knowledge is called "place," while freedom in relationships and without restraint is called "act abandonment." Bauman spent 20 years studying parental and newborn behaviour to determine how it influences children's growth and development. She articulated characteristics of parenting, such as attentiveness and demandingness that contribute to children's capacity for self-awareness and independent decision-making. In their quest for absolute control, what do parents really want? The term "demanding" is often used to describe parents who want absolute control. It was revealed that the frequency of interactions with parents was a reliable indicator of their level of attentiveness. It takes into account the children's individual strengths, aspirations, and emotional needs, as well as their accomplishments and the way they feel and act. The way a kid is raised in a family has a significant impact on his outlook on life and should be assumed to be the norm for most individuals in society. If a parent could always get away with cheating, a child who was never given anything would grow up thinking that dishonesty was commonplace and that anybody could get away with it. Being a mother is one of life's greatest trials, but it's also one of the most rewarding. Parental activities in the home have a substantial impact on children's social and emotional development, just as they do in other social and educational contexts.

Why Is Parenting Different

After reading about how different parenting styles may have a significant influence on a child's growth, you might find yourself wondering why all parents do not just use an authoritative parenting style. After all, this approach to raising children is the one that is most likely to result in children who are happy, confident, and competent. What are some of the possible explanations for the wide variety of parenting styles? Culture, personality, family size, parental history, financial class, educational level, and religious affiliation are only few of the many factors that might account for these disparities. The way in which individual parents choose to raise their children also contributes to the distinctive flavor that each and every family have. For instance, a woman may exhibit a parenting style that is more authoritative, while a father may choose an approach that is more permissive. It is necessary for parents to learn how to work with one another as they blend different aspects of their own parenting styles in order to produce an approach to parenting that is consistent and coherent.

Authoritative Versus Authoritarian Parenting

The words authoritative and authoritarian have a very similar tone. Both of Baumrind's parenting styles in psychology, authoritative and authoritarian, involve a position of power. Nonetheless, despite the fact that their titles are comparable, the underlying ideas and the impacts on children are very different. The following are the distinguishing qualities between authoritative parenting and authoritarian parenting styles.

- **Parental Warmth-** Parents who are authoritative are more likely to be loving, caring, and attentive than those who are authoritarian. Attachment theory, created by psychologist Mary Ainsworth in the 1970s, posits that a child's connection to their carers may be strengthened via responsive parenting. Secure bonds lead to better mental and physical wellness in children. Several investigations have shown that children raised by authoritative parents are happier than those raised by authoritarian ones. Children raised by authoritarian parents tend to have strong emotional regulation skills. In doing so, they strengthen their ability to bounce back fast from setbacks and build resilience. Authoritarian parents are the polar opposite of authoritative ones in terms of affection and attention. Authoritarian parents are emotionally distant and distant. They try to stifle kids' emotions because they see it as a sign of weakness.

- **Dom-** Autonomy and independence are encouraged in children raised by authoritative parents. They don't impose strict rules on their kids, but they do keep a careful eye on them and discipline them when necessary. The likelihood of a youngster engaging in antisocial conduct, delinquency, or drug misuse is drastically decreased when they are under their parents' watchful eye, according to (Dishion and Mahon, 1998).studies relationships that are warm and supportive between parents and their children are optimal for parental monitoring. Children of authoritative parents are often included in family decision-making processes. There should be two-way dialogue. Yet, authoritarian parents actively hinder their children from developing a sense of autonomy. Child participation in the decision-making process is not encouraged. Parental instructions are more like commands than pleas from the children.

- **Rules-** Each kind of parent, authoritative and authoritarian, is rigorous and has high standards for their children. When it comes to raising children, there are two types of authoritative parents: those who are rigorous but loving, and those who are strict but uncaring. Rules are discussed and explained by authoritative parents to their offspring. They're willing to have a give-and-take conversation and change the rules if necessary. We train our kids to obey without inquiry. Parents who are authoritative or authoritarian tend to be very rule-oriented. Their strategy is different. Parents that are very authoritarian tend to impose harsh restrictions on their children. When youngsters disobey their rules, they are met with severe punishment. There is no place for questioning or negotiating with children; they have to just obey orders. These rigid guidelines help them keep their youngster under control. The threat of punishment is used to maintain control over the children.

- **Control-** Authoritative parents, like authoritative ones, have strict rules and a tight rein on their children. The children of authoritarian parents, however, are also subject to strict psychological control. They have the self-assured conviction that they are the last arbiters of truth. Their offspring must always adhere to their standards of behaviour and value judgement. Most authoritarian parents seem to be concerned that they don't exert enough authority over their kids. For this reason, they want to do the exact opposite, although to an extreme degree, by becoming very authoritarian parents themselves. To maintain psychological control over their children, authoritarian parents play on their children's natural dread of them. When parents resort to psychological control as a form of punishment, they increase their children's likelihood of being compliant, fearful, and reliant. Some kids act out in negative ways like hitting and biting as a consequence of their struggle to break free from parental authority.

- **Discipline-** Authoritative parents often resort to time-outs and other forms of natural punishment rather than harsher methods. Parents that are more authoritarian tend to use harsher discipline methods. The interesting thing is that authoritative parents tend to have higher expectations than authoritarian parents, while allowing their children greater freedom and autonomy. They are also more reliable when it comes to carrying out the next action. While disciplining their children, authoritarian parents resort to severe methods. However, there are instances when they stop providing the kids with the help they formerly did. Moreover, there are others who resort to physical violence and/or verbal threats. Authoritative parents, on the other hand, tend to be more moderate when dealing with their offspring. That doesn't mean they're slacking off, however. Instead, parents explain to their kids about why it's necessary to take away some privileges or pleasures as a kind of punishment. Even dominant parents, who often have it together, get angry sometimes.

- **Effects On Kids-** The general outcomes for children improve when parents exercise authority. Nonetheless, other ethnic groups, such as Black Americans and Asian Americans, do show some academic performance variation. It's possible that kids of strict parents do better in school because they're held to higher standards and have clearer boundaries. High levels of parental participation in authoritative parenting have also been linked to high levels of academic success in children. Authoritative parents often help out at their kids' schools and keep a close eye on their children's homework. Parental participation has been shown to improve students' academic outcomes. On the other hand, authoritarian parents also set strict rules and expectations for their children. Several of them are also actively engaged in their kids' academic life. Authoritarian parents, on the other hand, exercise extreme psychological control and embrace harsh punishment as a means of child correction. Even if they do well in school, children with authoritarian parents are more likely to struggle emotionally and psychologically.

Changing Parenting Styles

In the past, parents played a central role in raising their children. That is, parents often raised their kids in a way that reflected their own priorities and ideals. But, as time has passed, a shift from a parent-centered to a child-centered perspective has taken place. For a long time, researchers in the field of human development relied on a straightforward parent effects model, which postulated that family impacts flowed only in one direction, from parents to their offspring. Yet, recent studies have shown that parents' parenting styles are affected by their children's actions. The impact that children have on their parents is highlighted by the "child effects" concept of the family. It's impossible to tell who has more of an impact when a kid's antisocial behaviour leads to a parent's resorting to a forceful and unsuccessful parenting style, and when that in turn leads to even more antisocial behaviour on the part of the child. The transactional model of familial influence is most suitable for developing this situation. Including two-way influences between parent and kid (Sigelman, 1999). We have adjusted the way that we parent to ensure that each of our children is raised in an atmosphere that fosters connection, a sense of safety, and love. This is a new approach for us, but I have discovered that it brings a great deal more pleasure to parenting, and as a result, our children are, for the most part, happier. The closer they are to us and the more they sense that we love them, the more they want to do all they can to make us happy. There are still a lot of disagreements and arguments amongst the children in our house, but there is a lot less shouting and spanking going on. And I really hope that our children are aware that they are loved no matter what happens.

Paternal Parenting

In the past, fathers' role as parents did not get a lot of attention, but in recent years, this perspective has received a lot more consideration. (Murray et al., 2014) Although some research suggest that the effects of both mother and paternal parenting are comparable, other studies have produced findings that are inconclusive (McGrath & Repetti, 2000). There have been a number of studies that have focused on either mother parenting or the scores of maternal and paternal parenting together (Rote & Smetana, 2016). The level of control exercised by fathers is an important factor to consider when attempting forecasting the deviant behaviours of children. The likelihood that adolescents would engage in internalising behaviours is reduced when their fathers provide warmth and control (Sekaran et al., 2020). When dads are present and actively involved in their children's development, it has a significant impact on a child's self-esteem, body image, moral standards, academic success, and social competence. This is because fathers tend to be more attentive to their children. Self-esteem, mental health, and overall happiness in life are all highly correlated with having a father figure in the home. There was a correlation found between authoritative parenting and lower levels of depression, as well as higher levels of self-esteem and overall life satisfaction. It is often believed that children suffer more negative effects from lenient female parenting than they do from permissive father parenting. Control exercised by parents is an essential factor in determining whether or not a kid will exhibit deviant behaviours.

A reduction in the likelihood of teenagers engaging in self-harming behaviours is associated with fathers who are warm and authoritative. There is a favourable correlation between the autonomy conferring attitude and attentiveness of dads and the well-being of their children, particularly teenagers. Children exhibited troublesome behaviour, particularly boys, when their fathers exercised a greater degree of paternal control over their lives. The amount of influence that dads have on their children is far lower than that of mothers, and their conflicts with their children are fewer and milder. On the other hand, these problems are said to be caused by dads due to the fact that fathers spend less time with their children. In their conversations with their children, fathers tend to centre the conversation on practical objectives. Children raised in homes where parents and children have positive, nurturing interactions tend to grow up to be successful adults who contribute positively to society. While an unpleasant parent-child connection formed as a result of an unfavourable parental attitude, which is linked to maladjustment and aberrant personality traits.

Parenting And Identity

The bond between parents and children is crucial because it determines how a kid will develop emotionally and behave in the world. This has repercussions for their mental, emotional, physical, and social health as well. So, a child's parents are in a position of authority and responsibility. Being the initial role models, they must keep a close eye on their charges and be there for them at all times. While every kid is unique and has his or her own set of skills, it is the parents who have the most potential to mold and guide their children. Encouraged children are less likely to be broken by setbacks since they are able to maintain a positive outlook no matter how difficult their situation may be. Adolescents usually acquire the social skills and competencies they exhibit in their peer group from their parents and other family members. Adolescents benefit much from supportive family relationships, but their own efforts are crucial as well. There has to be a lot of trying out different things, both professionally and personally, throughout this process.

While over the rest of his life, he will be polished, reevaluated, and take on new things, the identity he developed in adolescence will enable him adapt to and contribute to society, keeping a significant weight. Researchers have studied parenting methods and identity statuses (sometimes called "special identity planes") at length. According to Santrock (1995), adolescent identity development is affected by the parenting style of the parents. Acceptance of traditional values and the free expression of those beliefs constitute a mature identity. Adolescents need both the parental influence that instills conventional values and the peer influence that allows them to express themselves. Nonetheless, extreme fluency from adults and/or peers may impede teens' independent participation. So, the ways in which parents raise their children have an impact on their children's development and maturation.

Adolescents' identities are profoundly influenced by their parents. Successful parenting involves making the teenager feel safe, which in turn encourages the adolescent to think for themselves. Evidently, adolescence is a time in life when a person would rather rely on themselves than on their family on a psychological level. In reality, parents should encourage their teenager to explore his or her interests and take risks in order to facilitate the development of a unique sense of self. Therefore, coming into one's own and developing an identity are not solitary endeavours. Both the teenager and his or her parents play an important role in this process. It's crucial to assess whether or whether teenage identity is influenced by parental parenting style, and if so, to what extent. Finding the parenting style accountable for this impact is just as important as understanding the gender differences and the age variations within adolescence in identity development. Parents are included in this procedure because they work jointly to care for and discipline their children. By this process, the teenager will develop the ability to articulate his own perspectives. Students pick up on the importance of listening to others, valuing their opinions, and understanding that they are accountable for their own ideas.

Adolescents develop a sense of social competence, self-confidence, and social responsibility when they have a positive connection with their parents. All of these things would be unavailable to him in a relationship that lacked quality, which would undoubtedly have a detrimental impact on his or her ability to develop an independent sense of self and grow into an adult. Most families now struggle more than ever before to deal with the challenges posed by their teenagers. This disagreement may not have a detrimental impact on all families, but it will have a significant impact on 15-25% of families. It adds to the urge that teenage children have, which is to be away from their parents. Teenagers have the impression that their musical and fashion preferences are distinct from those of their parents at this point in their development. Researchers looked at different parenting techniques and eminences of identity as well as different identity planes. Their point of view is that the parenting techniques may be shown to have an impact on the level of identity accomplishment in teenagers. The key to developing a strong identity is learning to appreciate traditional values and expressing those beliefs in a manner that is authentic to you. In this sense, young people require the impact of both their parents and the influence of their peer group in order to be instructed in traditional values. It's possible that a lot of pressure from their parents and/or their peers will get in the way of their personal participation. So, parenting strategies have a greater impact on the development of an individual's identity throughout the teenage years. The relationship between parenting style and an adolescent's struggle with identity development occurs via the process of self-differentiation.

Teenage identity development is variables that are goal-oriented. Adolescents may only develop a healthy sense of identity if their parents foster free speech, tolerance for other points of view, and mutual respect. When parents use an emotionally-based parenting style, their children may exhibit identity-related problems including anger, restrictiveness, emotional distance, or a false sense of rejection. Parental binding behaviours, systemic rigidity, and discord in the family's capacity to adapt to the child's development into adulthood are all major impediments to the identity formation processes. These psychological and behavioural aspects of parenting are characteristic of the aforementioned styles and may either aid or impede teenagers in their quest for self-identity. Emancipation is a crucial problem in the evolution of the parent-adolescent relationship and is not merely something that happens to teenagers as they become older. As children reach their late teenage years, they must face the reality of separation from their parents when they leave home to pursue further education. There is a literal and figurative wall separating them. Teenagers often want to find their own identities apart from that of their parents and have attitudes and viewpoints that vary from those of their elders.

Adolescents' identity formation is influenced by a combination of three elements, including the parenting dimensions of acceptance/rejection, firm/lax control, and psychological autonomy/control. Individuals go through a process of identity formation in which they actively investigate and eventually adhere to their own unique morals, worldviews, and life goals. Parents who have an authoritarian parenting style set firm boundaries for their children and adolescents and discipline them when they violate those boundaries. Parents who have a permissive parenting style, on the other hand, are very accepting and affirming of their children and place very few demands on them. Authoritarian parenting styles are more common. Acceptance and affirmation play a role to some degree in the parenting methods of authoritative parents; yet, strict control is used while disciplinary measures are being carried out.

CHAPTER-2

ACADEMIC PROBLEMS AND ACADEMIC ACHIEVEMENT

The academic success of teenagers is significantly impacted by the assistance they get from their families. Each child's achievement in school is directly proportional to his or her feeling of safety and acceptance. A parent is a kid's first and most important instructor, which means that the home environment is where the youngster will get their first exposure to social interaction. A growing number of middle class and affluent parents are sending their children to boarding schools and private schools, in the belief that their children would thrive academically and socially in these environments. It has been shown that some parenting techniques, such as parental monitoring, are favorably correlated with academic achievements among adolescents from minority groups. Also, excellent parent–child connections have been linked to the academic success of young people from underrepresented groups (Alfaro et al., 2009). According to the integrative model of parenting developed by Darling and Stenberg (1993), the consequences of parenting techniques are somewhat dependent on the nature of the connection that exists between the parent and the kid. The emotional climate of the parent–child relationship was considered by Darling and Stenberg (1993) to be the overarching contextual variable in which parenting practices were carried out. Many variables may affect academic achievement, including sample demographic variables like gender, age, and socioeconomic position as well as variables like the caliber of classroom instruction and how children with special needs are organized. For instance, statistically speaking, pupils of a certain gender or race may often outperform their counterparts of a different gender or race in the classroom. The kid's academic success is influenced by a number of variables, including home, teacher, and student influences. Financial stress, working from home, family size, parenting style, and parental attitudes toward schooling are all home-related concerns. The connection between the instructor and pupils, in contrast, is tied to school variables since the teacher's attributes and skills have a big impact on how well children do.

The youngster may have trouble learning the fundamentals of education and interacting socially with teachers and classmates in a school setting. This may hinder cognitive growth, negatively affect language learning, and lead to maladaptive behavior patterns. On the other hand, parenting practices were defined as more specific behaviors that were tailored to the socialization domain of interest. It has been shown that parental monitoring is connected with a decrease in the number of minority students who drop out of school, as well as an increase in academic success, school engagement, and academic motivation. The degree to which parents are active in and supportive of their adolescents' school lives has a direct bearing on not just the adolescents' academic performance but also their personal and social development. A student's poor academic performance is a significant risk factor for dropping out of school. Separating the factors that affect students' grades has been a major focus of academic research. Dropout rates are often studied, although preschool and early care characteristics are seldom included. We searched for possible contributions to academic performance and the dropout process by reviewing the literature on the association between caregiver-child attachment and academic achievement, including attachment studies from the preschool years. Every child has the right to live with their biological family or with the person or people who can provide the greatest care for them, and to take part in all aspects of their community. Based on a survey of the relevant literature, we may infer that these families are made up of working professionals who place a high importance on education but who may be too preoccupied with their own life to take an active role in their children's day-to-day activities. They send their children to the top boarding schools so that they may feel secure leaving them in the care of someone they believe to be qualified to teach them while they are away. Parents also do this in other areas of their children's life, using the services and programs they pay for to provide their kids memorable experiences.

Researchers Kaisa, Hakan, and Jari-erik (2000) investigated the degree to which adolescent accomplishment strategies were linked to the parenting styles that were used in the household. According to the results, adolescents who came from authoritative homes used adaptive accomplishment methods. These techniques were distinguished by low levels of failure expectancies, task-irrelevant behavior, passivity, and self-enhancing attributions. In their turn, adolescents who came from households in which they were neglected used maladaptive tactics. These techniques were characterized by high levels of task-irrelevant behaviors, inactivity, and a lack of self-enhancing attributions. There is a favorable correlation between the participation of parents and their children's academic success. There was a negative correlation between authoritarianism and academic success. It was discovered that adolescents who came from families in which parents were working in low-income unskilled professions had lower levels of accomplishment than those adolescents who came from homes in which adults were worked in better earning occupations.

The word "achievement" refers to the state of having completed a task or a session with a positive result. Aspirations are realised in the satisfaction we experience upon achieving success. In this context, it refers specifically to one's level of mastery of a body of academic material. It includes how well they did on any class exams or quizzes. It's a method of finding out how much progress has been made in various academic areas. For this reason, academic success is crucial to a person's development. In this competitive world, it helps a youngster choose a career path. Competition in all walks of life is on the rise. The pressure to succeed in the classroom, on students, and on the educational system as a whole is exacerbated by the pursuit of excellence in the classroom. Students nowadays face intense pressure from their parents to succeed at the highest levels imaginable. The educational system is based on the student's performance in the classroom. Academic achievement, or how well a student conforms to institutional and governmental norms, is the benchmark by which schools are judged. Parents, lawmakers, and government education agencies all recognize that academic success is more critical in today's highly competitive job market. Much time and energy is spent on identifying, evaluating, tracking, and encouraging pupils' academic development since education is the sole path to success in the working world.

The only people who get to the top of society are the ones who have done well in school, as is common knowledge. All pupils are ranked on a scale from brilliant to mediocre to boring depending on their academic performance, and this ranking determines our fate. In addition, academic accomplishment refers to the acquisition of new information as well as improvements in one's ability to use such information in one's chosen field of study. The parent provides help to the kid by being authoritative and by responding to the child's needs with consistent, empathetic, and age-appropriate conduct. Raising a kid is different from parenting. Child rearing focuses on the process of teaching or bringing up a kid and the relationship between parent and child, whereas parenting highlights the roles and obligations of a parent and the attributes of a good role model. Regardless of whether or not they want to raise their children to be adults, most parents take care of their kids until they reach maturity by meeting their basic physical needs, keeping them safe from danger, and teaching them important life lessons. While animals often nvuture their young extensively, the process of raising a child typically takes less time and is less difficult. The typical adult of a species has a child-bearing capacity that is roughly inversely proportionate to the amount of time and energy the parents spend in raising them.

The parenting approach has an impact on academic performance. The very tiny percentage of pupils who come from households who are permissive underscores the significance of control and direction in attaining success. Parents have a key influence in their children's academic success by fostering a sense of agency and mastery in their children. Positive motivation, among other educational results, may be significantly impacted by the support of family members. To reinforce school lessons, encourage exploration and creativity, and develop children's special talents, Ferguson advises parents to establish clear and firm rules regarding homework, television watching, and other daily activities, and to actively seek out outside opportunities and extracurricular activities. There is a considerable inverse association between having an authoritarian parenting style and having successful academic children. There is a large and unfavourable association between an authoritarian parenting style and the professional route of the students, as well as a significant and negative relationship between educational achievement and career path of the students. A strong correlation may be seen between the types of parenting and the academic success of the teenagers. There is a considerable correlation between a father's level of education and his approach to parenting. There are a number of reasons why children who are raised in an authoritative home tend to do better in school. Parents that are more authoritative tend to take an active interest in their children's life and help them maintain a strong concentration on school.

They're more likely to keep the youngsters on track with their education and motivate them to do their best. Furthermore, these kids have a better chance of succeeding since their parents are ready to help them along the way. There is a medium-level meaningful relationship between parenting styles and a child's approach to learning, and a low-level meaningful relationship, in the positive direction, between parenting styles and a child's approach to avoiding learning. Authoritarian and overprotective parenting styles had the greatest influence on the former, while permissive and authoritarian attitudes had the greatest influence on the latter. The authors identified a weak but significant correlation between parenting approaches and both performance approach and performance avoidance orientation. Statistical analyses reveal a close relationship between authoritarian and overprotective parenting styles and these inclinations. The academic success and motivation of teenagers are significantly influenced by the parental style. According to research by Ling Pong et al. (2009), children whose parents take an authoritative stance are more likely to succeed academically. There are three explanations for why authoritative parenting is linked to academic success in high school. To begin, he said that parents who adopt an authoritative stance provide their kids with a feeling of serenity and independence while also helping them achieve academic achievement. Second, he said that authoritative parents show their kids the results of their actions.

Children benefit from explanations because they get a firm grasp of the values, wishes, and aims of their parents in the context of their educational experiences. Finally, he advocated for authoritative parents to have two-way communication with their children. Positive correlation between parents' participation and their children's academic success. According with the research, society at large and teachers in particular have blamed a lack of parental participation for a variety of educational issues. Parental aspiration/expectation for children's school accomplishment was shown to have the highest association with kids' academic achievement, while parental home supervision was found to have the least relationship, as determined by moderator analysis. When students' overall academic performance was used as an indication, rather than their performance in individual courses, the correlation was much greater. Maladaptive coping mechanisms, such as task-irrelevant behaviour, inactivity, and a lack of self-enhancing attributions, were often used by adolescents from neglectful households.

Turner (2009) compares the authoritarian approach to parenting to a military state. This is thus due to the fact that fast and unquestioning obedience to rules and directives is expected and required. Because of this, parental and child interaction becomes fake and mechanical. The kids aren't shown any love or care. The point is to be obedient and attentive. Such kids could have it hard because of this. Children in authoritarian households may do well in school because they are used to being held to a high standard. Sometimes, these kids may really shine in class, which is a typical observation. Such kids may achieve academic success but have a shy, reticent personality. Moore's (2011) research found that kids whose parents let them do anything they want outside of school led to a decline in academic performance. Although the aforementioned works stress the detrimental effects of permissive parenting on children's academic outcomes, this research argues that the two have no correlation. Parents who have authority over their kids back them up, push them to achieve well in school, and explain why that's important. That's why kids who grow up with strong adults in their lives tend to be healthier and more successful in school. Research has shown that different parenting styles are linked to different teenage motivation and success in school. A majority of research found a positive correlation between kids' perceptions of parental approval and their performance in school, whereas those of parental rejection were inversely connected (Uddin, 2011). The findings of this study indicate that the parent-child relationship of elementary school students is a negative predictor of academic pressure. This means that the stronger the parent-child relationship, the lower the level of academic pressure, which is in line with the majority of the findings from earlier research and provides additional support for the attachment theory and the pressure buffer model. It demonstrates that a healthy parent-child relationship is a protective factor for elementary students' academic pressure, which can be interpreted as follows: a healthy parent-child relationship is conducive to the establishment of active parent-child attachment and promotes parent-child communication and family support (Mulyadi et al., 2016).

Parents that fall into the authoritarian category tend to set very high demands for their children but provide little in the way of support or instruction to help them reach those goals. There's a chance they won't pay attention to their child's struggles in school and won't provide the supplementary resources necessary for them to succeed. The parents have an impact, both physically and mentally, on their children, which in turn has an effect on the children's growth and, in particular, their academic accomplishments (Yusup & Ahmad, 2016).

The primary emphasis of the authoritarian parenting style is on the parent imposing their norms without providing any explanation. An accepting parent is one who actively encourages their child's uniqueness, self-control, and self-assertion by responding positively to their child's wants and requests. Furthermore, a larger amount of parental psychological control was associated with lower levels of accomplishment, whereas a higher level of parental autonomy was associated with higher levels of success in school. It has been known for a long time that early childhood and the early school years are very important for adult well-being and success (Diniz et al., 2021). Education that is tailored to a child's stage of development from the beginning of their schooling leads to improved academic performance in subsequent years. In spite of the enormous number of research that has been conducted in this field, there is a significant lack of consensus about how parents should be conceived of and evaluated (Tazouti and Jarlégan, 2019). Some academics describe parental engagement as participation in extracurricular activities at their children's schools, while others define it as the parents' goals and aspirations for their children, and yet others define it as participation in their children's educational pursuits at home. Recent studies have shown that the idea of parental engagement is multifaceted, covering a broad variety of actions taken by parents in relation to their children's educational experiences. Researchers just lately came to this realisation. According to Epstein, parents' participation in their children's schooling evolves throughout time. Rather, variations in any one of three overlapping spheres of influence—the family, the community, and the school—can affect the ways in which parents are involved. Family ties play an essential role in a child's development (Popa, 2022). What defines a parent's child care attitude is how they interact with their kid, from how they greet them to what they expect from them to how they talk to them to how they discipline them. We accept the child's destructive conduct because the parents feel unable to stop him or her. Although they may be better at caring for their children, these parents often struggle to keep their kids in check. Their lack of discipline and low expectations for their children stems from the fact that they offer them too much leeway.

Authoritarian parents exert an unhealthy amount of control over their children by enforcing rigid rules and restrictions. What's important to such parents isn't whether or not their kids like them, but rather that they behave properly and respect authority without question. In spite of their track record of child-rearing failures, these parents still consider themselves to be the most authoritative figures in their kids' lives. Children who had parents who were authoritative tended to perform better in school because of the child-centered relationship and open communication that they had with their parents. This is because these children were more likely to get the additional assistance and direction that they might require. Authoritarian parents, on the other hand, set greater expectations for their children but did nothing to support them in developing the skills necessary to meet those expectations. When the kid misbehaves, they punish it with words and sometimes with physical punishment, but they never acknowledge the good they see (Song et al., 2022).

This refers to a parenting approach in which parents have excessively high standards for their children (Ren and Zhu, 2022). These parents are the most set in their ways and also the ones that make snap judgements. Finally, authoritative parents help their kids through words and touch. They care deeply for and are very attached to their young. Such parents take a more collaborative approach with their young children. They have high hopes because they know their children can achieve them. They're trying to teach their kids to be kind and helpful. They pay attention to their kids and treat them with kindness and understanding because of this (Liu et al., 2022). Most people agree that authoritative parenting is the optimal approach to raising children, but the standards by which good parents should be judged are not hidden or obscured. Its flexible design makes it easy to alter its appearance. Children's relationships with their families are critical to their growth (Popa, 2022). Bowlby's theories were validated, in particular when applied to the problem of parental-attachment and its consequences on the academic performance of elementary school children who are sent away for the school year. Although attachment issues have shown to have far-reaching consequences on a child's development, it is puzzling that parents should take the lead in sending their children to boarding schools or institutions when their children are still in elementary school.

Parental child care attitudes are defined by the parents' warm and caring approach to the child; expectations of the child; communication with the child; and disciplinary attitudes toward them. When parents follow the approach of permissive parenting, they give their children the freedom to behave whatever they choose without questioning the motivations behind their child's actions. We accept the child's destructive conduct because the parents feel unable to stop him or her. Although they may be better at caring for their children, these parents often struggle to keep their kids in check. Their lack of discipline and low expectations for their children stems from the fact that they offer them too much leeway. There is a strong correlation between how parents raise their kids and how successful they are in school, according to several studies. The majority of studies have shown that parental participation in their children's education is good for the kids. Several studies with elementary school pupils have shown a correlation between parental involvement and improved academic performance, student happiness, school attendance, homework completion, and educational aspirations.

The results showed that parental involvement had a favourable effect on students' grades, homework completion rates, school attitudes, and the likelihood that they would drop out of high school. Several studies have demonstrated that parental participation in their children's education is positively correlated with their children's academic outcomes, including increased school engagement, better homework habits, less absenteeism and truancy, and higher grades. Despite the fact that the affects of parents on their children's accomplishment objectives have only lately been investigated, these goals are a crucial motivating aspect for comprehending kids' involvement and learning. Generally speaking, the research found that parental control was linked to performance objectives, whereas parental engagement or autonomy was connected with mastery goals. Due to its strong correlation with mastery-approach objectives, parental acceptance was linked with a favourable learning profile, including high success. In addition, performance-avoidance objectives linked parental control to a poor academic profile, particularly low accomplishment. These results provide credible factual backing to the idea that pupils' success is influenced by both their parents' and their own aspirations for them. Adolescents whose parents exhibited permissive parenting methods had worse academic attainment than their peers for a variety of reasons, including but not limited to reduced motivation to learn.

Parents that choose a liberal parenting approach give their kids complete freedom to decide how they will behave and act. Parents are increasingly apathetic and seldom participate in the critical choices that teenagers make. Teenagers from very liberal environments are thus likely to lack clear standards and expectations for high accomplishment, which may ultimately result in low desire for effort and subpar academic performance. Authoritarian parents often engage in strict and extensive supervision of their children. Children and teenagers might lose motivation if they are constantly monitored.

Parents who gave their kids a lot of freedom were less likely to be invested in helping them succeed in school. This kind of parent is likely to take a "hands-off" approach to their child's education and let them figure things out on their own. They seem emotionally detached from their kids, and they don't set as many limits for them. If you look at the children's grades, you'll see that they tend to be lower. Children with permissive parents fared better in school than those of negligent parents. This would be the case because permissive parents, although providing little care, would still be preferable than absentee ones. The educational results of children raised by permissive parents were better than those of children raised by negligent parents. This would be the case because permissive parents, although providing little care, would still be preferable than absentee ones. On the issue of inattentive parenting in regards to education, they paid little attention to their children, who had the worst academic outcomes. Children of these parents may have believed they didn't have to put in any effort in school since they weren't given any direction. Furthermore, they lacked a protector or a motivator to prioritise academic achievement on their behalf. Parents who take an interest in their children's schooling and create a positive atmosphere at home for learning have a significant impact on their children's sense of self-efficacy, which in turn improves their academic performance. It is essential to take into consideration the effects of various parenting methods on the developmental result of teenagers, as this will ensure a successful future for them. When all of the aforementioned research is taken into consideration, it is possible to draw the conclusion that an authoritative parenting style results in a number of positive developmental outcomes in adolescents. This is because an authoritative parenting style involves parental monitoring and supervision, which increases an adolescent's exposure to positive activities and decreases the teen's opportunities for engaging in risky behaviours and delinquent activities. A parenting style that is warm but yet firm enables teenagers to be autonomous within the context of restrictions and boundaries that are developmentally appropriate for their age.

CHAPTER-3

PARENTAL STYLE AND ITS CORRELATE

The way in which parents interact with their offspring is important for a variety of reasons. From the parents' point of view, these goals include moral and psychological education, talent and skill discovery and development, and acculturation to societal norms and expectations. Having a strong family unit is essential as a foundation for any healthy society. Young people are impacted by their families and communities more than by their peers and the wider community. The creative, cultural, social, and moral developments of a kid are profoundly impacted by parental involvement. One aspect affecting the physical and emotional well-being of children is the quality of their relationships with their parents. During the current topic, an extensive literature review is conducted on parenting behaviour, the father's and mother's roles in the context of a child's development and wellbeing, parental involvement, the dimensions and styles of parenting and their association with the various aspects of a child's life, and the significant outcomes during adolescence and early adulthood. It is reasonable to anticipate that the child's psychological and social development would be affected differently by the various parenting styles due to the vital role that parental behaviour training plays in the creation of a child's character and the social environment.

The constant attitude that parents have towards their children is reflected in their parenting styles, which are in turn founded on particular attitudes and patterns of conduct. This encompasses the myriad of interactions and strategies that parents use in an effort to mould the long-term development of their children. Many parenting habits are risk factors for a child's mental health, and others have a long-lasting influence on a child's development, so it's important to be aware of how you parent. Having children may be a catalyst for personal growth, self-assurance, and happiness. Being a parent means taking on new challenges, which is great because it gives kids a chance to develop and show off their skills in new ways. Parents and children provide each other immense and lasting joy (Bornstein, 2001). Although raising children is mostly an individual experience, it also has significant societal implications. To parent is to do it within the framework of a particular family. There are strong sentimental bonds that keep some relatives close. There is still a dearth of research on the relationship between parenting styles and teenage suicide conduct, with the majority of the literature coming from high-income nations. With the aim of enhancing the data about potential risk or protective variables for teenage suicide conduct, parenting techniques, beyond the well-known four parenting styles, and youth suicidal behaviour have been studied. This might also serve as a basis for conceptualising and evaluating the effectiveness of treatments aimed at reducing suicide behaviour in this population. Such a loose set of parent's exhibit strong responsiveness and empowerment in the relationship with their offspring, at the same time having very little to no influence it has also been argued that gender may play a role in whether or not parenting correlates with the child's anxiety. Parenting can have greater impacts on girls in the middle and earlier ages than for these two groups, although infant fear has a greater impact on boys during puberty. To be in line with what had been predicted, the greater amount of parental opposition and strictness was related to the higher levels of children's anxiety. In keeping with previous research on child anxiety and authority, it follows that this is the amount of power that parents have over their children. Anxiety in children has been connected to their parents' parenting styles, including warmth, rejection, (over)protection, and nervous behavior. There is a substantial correlation between overprotective parenting (a pattern of intrusive governance and concomitant restraint put on the child's behaviors) and poor warmth (responsiveness) in the home. Families where there is a lack of warmth and support, where parents lack behavior management skills, and where children's lives are marked by conflict or maltreatment have been linked to an increased risk of delinquency, while loving and nurturing families can shield children even from a dangerous and damaging outside world. Authoritative parenting was shown to be the most effective method of raising children, whereas authoritarian and neglectful parenting was found to have a positive correlation with juvenile criminality. It was also shown that preteen years were fertile times for criminal behavior.

Parenting Style And Mental Health

Adverse mental health conditions account for a disproportionate share of the worldwide illness burden experienced by teenagers and have far-reaching consequences. Substantial societal costs are associated with mental health issues. It's no secret that many kids and teens are struggling with mental health issues. The necessity for preventative measures is emphasised by experts in the field and by government health agencies. Moreover, adolescent mental illness is a contributing factor to risky conduct. Acceptance and rejection by parents, who are often children's primary attachment figures, may have profound consequences on their development and well-being. More specifically, good parenting styles, such parental emotional warmth, have a beneficial influence on adolescents' mental health, whereas negative parenting styles, like rejection, have a detrimental and long-lasting effect on adolescents' mental health. Yet, family systems theory argues that a child's mental and emotional development is profoundly impacted by the overall strength, harmony, and well-being of his or her family. There are several elements that might contribute to the onset of mental health issues in young people. One such factor that has a direct effect on a person's psychological well-being is the parenting style they were raised with.

Mental health is largely determined by the quality of the parent-child connection and the parenting practices in place. A variety of studies have shown that parenting practices, family dynamics, and relationships all have an impact on children's emotional well-being. Communicating with one's children is the single most important aspect of every parenting approach. Studies have shown that parents who use an authoritative approach have a positive effect on their children's mental health. Authoritative parenting was shown to be linked to better mental health, whereas authoritarian parenting was found to have no effect on children's well-being. To a lesser extent than in a culture that values generosity; authoritarian parenting may have negative effects in an autocratic society. The degree to which a child's cerebral palsy worsens and the quality of their life after diagnosis are significantly impacted by their parents' parenting styles. According to the research conducted by Tiwari and Verma (2013), perceived paternal psychological support was shown to be a significant predictor for the majority of mental health disorders. According to research conducted by Vora (2013), favourable opinions of parenting are associated to improved, positive results in terms of a child's mental health and social maturity. This not only underscores the important role that parents play in assisting their children in more successfully integrating their personal and social lives, but it also offers up options for effective treatments when it comes to working with teenagers. Due to the inherent importance of the parent-child bond, the issue of whether or not positive interactions between parents and their offspring improve the latter's well-being is essential to resolve.

Adolescent alcohol use, school absences, and truancy are all decreased as a result. It also serves as a predictor of academic grades and is linked to greater levels of education; therefore it may help mitigate the detrimental effects of stress on health. In reality, their mental health and ability to complete activities are compromised, which slows down development and has negative effects. Childhood and teenage mental health problems may be exacerbated by psychosocial stress brought on by a dysfunctional home environment. The parent-child bond is the family's most crucial subsystem. The dynamics of the family are profoundly affected by the parenting style of the parents. Because our entire thought process occurs in the mind, ideas originate in the mind, and all types of directions are issued from the mind, which guide, conduct and behaviour as well as shape and regulate communication, determine personal and social functioning as well as adjustment, mental health is an essential part of one's overall health. Emphasis is placed on both subjective well-being and objective success in life as measures of positive mental health (Gilmour, 2014). A condition of positive mental health may be defined as an ever-evolving sense of fulfillment in which a person realises his or her full potential. Consciousness of one's own and other people's inherent value and worth. This person is not only able to function normally under the pressures of daily life, but is also effective in the workplace and has a positive impact on their community (Shilpa, 2014).Those who are thriving in life have a high sense of well-being, report often experiencing happy feelings, and are able to effectively navigate their psychological and social environments.

On the other hand, languishing refers to a condition of mental illness characterised by feelings of hopelessness, apathy, and disinterest in one's surroundings. Enjoyment of life, resilience in the face of setbacks, hopefulness in the face of adversity, the capacity to realise one's potential, and a feeling of belonging to a community are all components of mental health that may be contextualised in a variety of ways. Hence, one's mental wellness is crucial to his or her overall health and happiness (Sankar, Wani &Indumathi, 2017). There has been a growing recognition over the past few decades of the importance of mental health as a separate but interrelated aspect of overall health, as evidenced by recent studies from a variety of countries showing that those with the highest incidence and prevalence of mental illness also have the highest health priorities related to mental illness. Feeling good about oneself and having a positive outlook on life, having positive relationships with loved ones, being physically active and eating a balanced diet, having the ability to unwind and get enough sleep, and being involved and feeling a sense of belonging in one's community are all indicators of positive mental health.

Uninvolved parents have the expectation that their children will bring themselves up. They do not invest a significant amount of time or effort into satisfying the fundamental requirements of the children. It is possible for uninvolved parents to be negligent, although this is not always the case. It's possible that a parent who struggles with mental illness or addiction to substances, for instance, won't be able to meet all of their child's physiological or psychological requirements on a regular basis (Amy, 2019).

Parenting styles that are both authoritative and authoritarian have been shown to strongly predict emotional intelligence. Emotional IQ was not strongly predicted by permissive parenting. Although authoritarian and permissive parenting styles were both significant predictors of psychological suffering, the authoritative parenting style did not substantially predict psychological distress. Parenting style affects both psychological wellness and emotional intelligence. Given that adolescence is one of the most sensitive and significant periods of life, psychologists and theorists emphasise the importance of parents and parenting methods. However, very little research has been done on the relationship between parenting practices and a child's psychological pathology. While teenagers are affected by their surroundings and society, their families have a far greater impact on them since this is the first institution where their personalities are created. Children's moral, cultural, and social development may be highly influenced by their families. One of the important aspects in determining how well-adjusted and healthy a teenager is raised is their family. The act of caring for and educating one's own children on a daily basis is known as parenting. The ways in which parents raise their children have both long-term and short-term effects on their children's development and these effects extend to the children's physical, emotional, and mental health. It has a crucial function in the development of pediatric mental illnesses as well as in the maintenance of such diseases.

The way in which children are raised may be characterised in a number of different measurable categories by the parenting style (Sahithya, et, al, 2019). Early childhood experiences that are linked to parenting, such as low levels of parental warmth, rejection, and inconsistent parenting, are tied to insecure attachment and negative emotions in children, both of which have been identified as risk factors for subsequent suicidal behaviour. One research demonstrated the curved link between overprotective parenting and suicide ideation; that is, overprotective parenting can only minimise suicidal ideation up to a certain point and beyond that point, it may have negative effects on suicidal conduct (Arafat, et, al, 2020). Early childhood experiences that are not linked to parenting have not been found to be associated with suicidal behaviour (Zortea,et,al, 2021).This is not the case, and many parents are oblivious to the influence they have on their children despite the fact that they have this ability. The absence of educational opportunities is the root cause of this predicament. The emotional resources that parents need to effectively raise their children and prepare them for life in this world are not readily available to them. There is not just a lack of abilities, but also a lack of emotional intelligence and mental stability. Those parents who are detrimental to their children's overall development often suffer with their own mental health difficulties as well as drug misuse or dependence. This may have a negative impact on their ability to parent effectively.

According to the opinions of those who work in mental health, they victimise themselves. Obviously, parents who deal with these kinds of problems won't be able to or won't be able to attend to the requirements of their children. In terms of their academic performance, emotional well-being, psychological health, and the capacity to interact effectively with others. Children are placed in foster care when they have been neglected or mistreated by their mentally unstable parents, placed in residential treatment institutions, confinement centres, or juvenile prisons for an extended length of time, or when they have been incarcerated for an extended period of time. One may consider them to be victims of other victims. As a consequence of this, individuals end themselves in undesirable situations such as prostitution, drug addiction, sociopathic and criminal behaviour, mental health concerns or emotional messes. Arafat, et, al, (2022) found that authoritarian parenting style has been linked to suicide conduct in adolescents as well as later in life, suggesting a connection between the two. In order to properly evaluate the connection, further research using sound methodology is required. This specific review found evidence to support the hypothesis that authoritarian parenting and the neglect of children throughout childhood have a connection to suicidal conduct during adolescence and later in life.

Parenting Style And Emotional Intelligence

It's generally agreed that the parent-child interaction is crucial for a child's development of an emotional intelligence. A number of studies have shown contemporaneous and longitudinal connections between children's conversations of emotions with parents and their knowledge of emotions, highlighting the importance of discussing emotions with parents early on. Nonetheless, there is considerable variation among parents in terms of how openly they express their own feelings with their offspring. Children with confident parents may have more opportunity to talk about and reflect on their own emotions since their parents are more likely to open up about both good and negative feelings. The hallmark of a healthy connection is honest, open dialogue between parents and their children about their feelings. Everyone experiences a wide range of feelings. Because of its central significance in interpersonal communication, character formation, and thought processes, emotion has become an inevitable topic for psychologists, theorists, and developmental researchers alike. Emotional intelligence is defined as the ability to manage one's own emotional states. Parents have a profound effect on their children's emotional and social development, and studies on the topic have proven that the home is the first and most important place of learning for kids. The warmth of one's parents has a more significant effect on their children's emotional intelligence. Such a result is to be anticipated given the affectionate character of emotional intelligence. Perceived warmth has the most important function in the development of emotional intelligence, however having some degree of autonomy is crucial. By meeting their kid's demand for affection, parents may inadvertently provide their child the drive and energy he needs to develop the skills essential for self-regulation and emotional competence later in life. In this context, the self-determination theory (Deci & Ryan, 1985), a motivational model, suggests that when parents meet their children's basic needs, their children are better able to internalise their values and grow up with strong competencies in areas like self-appraisal, self-awareness, and emotion regulation.

The capacity of the parents to fulfill, to generate motivation, and to create internalised rules might help explain the impacts of parenting, such as warmth, on a child's emotional development. This skill aids the youngster in evaluating, controlling, and articulating his or her feelings. The youngster will demonstrate incompatibility if he adopts his parent's dysfunctional behavior-regulating routines in order to use them to manage his emotions. On the other side, if these habits of thought are effective, they may boost a kid's EQ and social skills. It appears from our findings that parents should begin their relationships with their children with a focus on warmth; and as the child matures and enters adolescence, these warm relationships should be complemented by recognition of emotions, thoughts, and choices, as well as permission of autonomy, in order to lead to reinforcing the child's capacity for self-confidence, self-initiation, self-regulation, and the experience of feeling emotionally whole. So, it is reasonable to suppose that parents' attitudes and practices have a major part in shaping their children's emotional intelligence. Nonetheless, there is a dearth of studies in this field. Emotional intelligence is a popular topic for study, and most studies have looked at how various parenting approaches affect their offspring's emotional intelligence (Fonte, 2009). The results showed a negative association between the permissive and authoritarian styles and emotional intelligence, with neglect being the most detrimental. The authoritative style (especially the control aspect) was shown to be the most potent predictor of emotional intelligence. Moreover, warmth is linked to better emotional intelligence, as well as better emotional management and use. There is a lack of adequate research on the connection between emotional intelligence and parental participation and autonomous support, especially in late adolescence.

Children may develop emotional and social competence, responsibility, independence, and confidence when they have a strong attachment to and open line of communication with their parents, who set clear expectations for behaviour. Parenting has a crucial influence in a child's growth and development in all areas, from the physical to the emotional to the social to the intellectual, from infancy to adulthood. The aim of this study was to examine the literature on children's emotional intelligence and to determine whether or not various parenting styles and parental training predict emotional intelligence similarly or differently from how they predict other developmental outcomes. So, it's clear that being a parent requires a high level of emotional intelligence. All people experience a wide range of emotions. Because of its central significance in interpersonal communication, personality development, and even cognitive processes, emotion has become an inevitable issue for psychologists, theorists, and developmental researchers alike. Emotional intelligence is defined as the ability to manage one's own emotional states. Several prior researches attempted to determine whether or not there was a connection between parenting methods and emotional intelligence. Many studies have examined parents' responses and behaviours in response to their children expressing their emotions, with consistent findings that parental attachment and emotional intelligence are directly related to one another. A research that looked at how people's perceptions of their parents' parenting influenced their own emotional intelligence revealed a favourable correlation between the two. Maternal warmth and encouragement of independence are two indicators of a person's emotional intelligence. The method in which parental affection is seen may be one of the most important variables in shaping a child's emotional intelligence. The results showed that high emotional intelligence was positively associated with an affectionate restricted parenting style, and negatively associated with an affectionless control or neglectful parenting style.

Adolescents whose parents shown a pattern of loving restriction were more likely to have high emotional intelligence than those whose parents displayed a pattern of neglect, and vice versa. The method in which parents punish their children has far-reaching and long-lasting effects on the development of the child's emotional life. Both severe treatment and sympathetic understanding have consequences. Existing research on parental attitudes towards their offspring reveals a wide spectrum of responses, from cold indifference to overt displays of affection. Several studies have shown that the home is a child's first and most significant learning environment, and that parents have a significant impact on their children's emotional and social development. Parents may assume a great deal of responsibility for moulding their children's emotional intelligence via their own attitudes and actions. Yet, research in this area is lacking. Children of moms who spend more time with them and engage in meaningful activities with them are more emotionally developed than those of mothers who spend less time with them. Parenting styles have an effect on children's emotional intelligence, with authoritarian and disciplinarian techniques having a detrimental impact. Instead, more democratic parenting was associated with better adaptation. The father's authoritative parenting style was significantly positively correlated with the goal-corrected partnership and only tangentially negatively correlated with emotional control. Emotional intelligence may be predicted in large part by either childhood abuse or parental connection.

Past research has shown that those who were victims of childhood abuse have greater trouble articulating their feelings and making accurate judgements about events and others. Reduced emotional intelligence is one of the many harmful effects of childhood abuse. Victimized children may be hesitant to talk about their feelings, and they may incorrectly interpret the emotions of others as threats (Schimmenti, 2017). Priya and Jaswanti's research from 2020 found that there is a significant positive association between different parenting styles and emotional intelligence in their study's findings. The researchers Peng et al. (2022) discovered that emotional intelligence, childhood abuse, and parental connection were all connected to one another. Mistreatment in childhood may result in feelings of insecurity and poor connection to one's parents. The building of healthy, personal connections is disrupted throughout childhood when a person is subjected to abuse, which may result in an insecure attachment.

Parenting Style And Self Esteem

There is no one parenting approach that is superior to all others since culture, environment, and individual characteristics are all unique to each child. It has been proved time and time again that a negative correlation exists between low levels of acceptance and high levels of over protectiveness in parenting styles and poor levels of self-esteem in children. Authoritarianism is characterised by this affectionless control, and the parenting style is thought to be related with social ineptitude and poor communication skills. This is because authoritarianism is characterised by this affectionless control.

Poor parenting, which may include a lack of parental care and warmth, was shown to be substantially related with low self-esteem and low life satisfaction, both of which can contribute to poor psychological well-being. A person's low sense of self-worth can result from a number of different factors, including but not limited to: unsupportive parents or influential role models, friends who are negative influences, a traumatic or otherwise emotionally trying life event, mood disorders, anxiety, or chronic physical health problems. Self-esteem is important because of its role in healthy human development. How a child acts and thinks as they grow up is influenced by their surroundings. A youngster learns from his parents and takes on their characteristics as his own as he grows up. Self-esteem is an important foundation for a child's growing identity and is profoundly shaped by the attitudes and actions of his or her parents. Someone's self-esteem isn't only a reflection of their beliefs; it also incorporates their overall view of themselves and the importance they place on themselves. Self-esteem significantly affects how we connect with our family members on a daily basis. One won't be able to fulfill their obligations to other family members if they feel horrible about themselves. This vicious spiral keeps on because the worse they feel about themselves, the worse they will treat one another and the more it will lower their self-esteem. Self-esteem is essential for self-identification, as well as for success in both personal and professional spheres.

According to Nijhof and Engels (2007), an authoritative parenting style is strongly associated with a child's good psychological and social development throughout adolescence. In contrast to the more authoritarian style of parenting, the permissive parent is warm and accepting of their child's ideas and interests. Children raised in a more relaxed, permissive environment have better self-esteem than those raised in a stricter, authoritative one (Martinez & Garcia, 2008). More specifically, previous research shows that parents who are loving and supportive may help their children develop higher levels of self-esteem (Yang & Liang, 2008). This remark suggests that the link between parenting methods and children's sense of self-worth requires further study. This is due in large part to the fact that children raised with an authoritative style of parenting tend to be more independent, have greater self-esteem, and learn to cope with stressful situations using ways that work for them (Hesari and Hejazi, 2011) Conflicts between parents and their adolescents arise as a result of the generation gap between them and their adolescents and the inability of parents to understand their adolescents, as Deshpande and Chhabriya (2013) found in their study of parenting styles and their effect on adolescents' self-esteem. Parental acceptance or support is positively associated to adolescents' self-esteem, and they found that adolescents who perceived an accepting attitude from their parents had better self-esteem than those who perceived an avoidance or concentration attitude from their parents. Yet since teenagers see their parents as their caretaker and occasionally defender, even minor punishment from parents may result in good self-esteem.

The self-esteem message might be favourable or negative. When someone's self-talk is upbeat and encouraging, it's a sign that they value themselves and have a balanced perspective on which they are. And those with low self-esteem focus on their flaws and shortcomings more often than their strengths and achievements. Hence, one's self-esteem may be seen as one's view on life, one's evaluation of oneself, and one's estimation of one's own worth. Researchers Hong, et, al (2015) looked at the link between parents' parenting styles and their children's levels of self-esteem. Students at universities with high self-esteem tend to come from families where the parents practice a liberal parenting style. There was also a substantial correlation between the way parents raised their children and their children's levels of self-esteem in college. The findings also showed that a student's self-esteem was positively related to an authoritarian parenting style, whereas it was negatively related to a permissive or authoritative one. Adolescents' levels of self-esteem were shown to increase when mothers exhibited more authoritative traits, according to research by Milu and Fathima (2015). Characteristics of authoritative parenting, such warmth and nurturing have been linked to positive effects on children's mental health and their ability to form satisfying connections with others.

Adolescents' perceptions of their parents' permissiveness did not correlate significantly with their own sense of self-worth. That's to be expected, given the teens' overall impression of their parents' permissiveness. There is a significant lack of study on the topic of parenting techniques and how they affect teenagers' sense of self-worth in Africa, despite the fact that this topic has received considerable attention in the literature with respect to western and Asian cultures. Few studies have looked at the relationship between parenting methods and teenagers' self-esteem; those that have done so have mostly focused on other outcomes. In a permissive home, parents set little limits on their children's behaviour. Indulgent, tolerant, unconventional, and receptive, yet not demanding or controlling (Garcia and Santiago, 2017). Parents who are more permissive tend to be more nurturing and accepting of their children but less strict in their expectations for behaviour. They tend to be overly accepting and kind, and if a child's choice doesn't endanger their safety, they usually go along with it. Children who are raised by authoritative parents are more likely to achieve optimal long-term health, happiness, and development. They are less likely to have mental health issues, interpersonal conflicts, or drug misuse, and they do better in school. They also tend to have fewer behavioural, emotional, and drug use issues, better academic outcomes, and more creative problem-solving skills (Banstola, et, al, 2020). Adolescents' feelings of connection to their parents might be affected by their parents' parenting practices. Insecure attachment, which may be further subdivided into attachment anxiety and attachment avoidance, is associated with having a troubled childhood (Kawamoto, 2020). Anxiety over being abandoned and a lack of emotional support from attachment figures may contribute to a poor self-perception, which in turn can lead to attachment disorder. Adolescents with high attachment anxiety tend to have poor self-esteem because they feel unworthy of receiving love and compassion. On the other side, those who struggle with attachment avoidance may be the ones who have a distorted view of how much their loved ones care about them. Low self-esteem is a common trait among those who struggle with attachment avoidance.

Szkody et al. (2021) conducted a meta-analysis and showed that children entering adolescence who were raised by authoritative or permissive parents reported more happiness and self-esteem than those reared by authoritarian parents. Even if just one parent (father or mother) is authoritative or permissive, this effect will remain. Moreover, teenage children whose parents exhibit both permissive and authoritarian parenting have much worse self-esteem. It's impossible to understate how much of an impact parents have on their children's development and happiness. The effects of parents' actions on their children's growth and development may be either beneficial or detrimental. The parenting approach used, in addition to other factors, will inevitably produce a certain result. A child's behaviour and academic performance might be affected by the parenting style that was used. It is well established that a child's success in developing healthy self-esteem is strongly influenced by the parenting style of his or her primary careers. One of the factors that have been researched extensively in relation to human development is parental style. Some researchers have shown that it is a strong predictor of a child's later success. The family, and particularly the parents' parenting techniques, may have a profound effect on a child's sense of self-worth. This is not to argue that parents directly affect their children's self-esteem, but rather that their parenting style has a "predisposing" influence on their children's self-esteem.

Parenting Style And Depression

A substantial body of research has revealed that the degree to which individuals who suffer from depression think that their parents did not give enough support for them and overprotected them when they were children. There is a link between perceived family disapproval and total adolescent stress, and if previous study can be accepted, there is a possibility that an individual may develop both the former and the latter. Two major aspects of parental behavior—rejection and control—have garnered attention throughout the vast body of research on parenting and juvenile psychopathology. In the literature, rejection is characterized as a set of parent behaviors that are indicative of indifference and dislike toward the kid (Clark and Ladd, 2000). Patients with depression are more likely to recall their parents as uncaring and overprotective, according to clinical research. Evidence from a variety of studies, including those including both clinically anxious and non-referred kids, shows a moderate relationship between parental control and rejection on one end of the continuum and juvenile anxiety on the other. The role of a parent in providing guidance and exercising excessive power Parents have a very low level of trust in their children, seem to advocate limited interaction with their children, and consistently exercise careful surveillance. It has been shown that the quality of the parent-child connection, specifically the degree of attachment or closeness that exists between the parent and the kid, has an impact on the behavioural and emotional well-being of children and adolescents (Liu, 2006). The data is very solid that children with more insecure attachments to their parents are more likely to exhibit severe behavioural issues and violent behaviour, as well as an increased risk of developing emotional troubles, including depressed and anxious symptomology (Allen, et al., 2007).

Nevertheless, in terms of the most detrimental behaviours, a considerable number of researches agreed with the distancing and dynamics studies that had been carried out, which had judged violence and verbal domination to be the most restrictive. Labovit's (2015) research sought to quantify and characterise teenagers' perceptions of their parents' parenting methods, as well as to examine the connections between these perceptions and depressive symptoms in young people. Results from a correlation study showed a significant link between authoritative parenting and less depressed symptoms. Parents who were permissive and moderately connected with depression in adolescents raised at a young age, but who were negative and strongly correlated with depression in adolescents raised in a loving environment, were discovered. They also found that children of either dominant or control-type parents did not show more signs of depression than those of permissive parents. The scores for mothers' excessive monitoring were shown to be substantially correlated with the involvement of child welfare agencies. Two parents' parenting styles may combine to generate a family's overall style, which can be authoritative, authoritarian, indulgent, or uninvolved depending on how the children rate their parents and how much involvement they get in their lives. In a research that was carried out by Nikoogoftar and Seghatoleslam (2015), the authors investigated the influence that parenting styles have in determining the likelihood of behavioural and emotional issues in teenagers. This study consisted of three different types of research: descriptive, correlational, and cross-sectional. According to the findings, an authoritarian parenting style is linked to a variety of mental health issues, including depression, behavioural issues, and emotional issues (total score). The authoritarian parenting style, on the other hand, has been linked to a number of mental health issues, including anxiety and depression, as well as behavioural and emotional issues. In addition, a link was found between permissive parenting styles and behavioural issues in children. The researchers came to the conclusion that their findings were in line with the findings of other studies that placed an emphasis on the role that parents play in forecasting the behavioural and emotional issues that children may have.

Children with at least one authoritative parent had far lower rates of depression and criminal behaviour. 11% of the variation in teenage depression might be attributed to differences in parenting styles. Better results were shown when children had one authoritative parent and either another authoritative or indulgent parent, or two indulgent parents, compared to when the mother was uninvolved and the father were either indulgent or uninvolved. The disparity between parents' and teachers' views of children's externalising (but not internalising) behaviour was strongly linked to poor parental acceptance of the kid. Parental perceptions of their children's internalising and externalising behaviour difficulties decreased with higher levels of parental engagement. Recent research has shown a correlation between parental sadness, and more specifically mother depression, and greater reports of behavioural and emotional issues in children. Early trauma was more likely to occur if dads did not provide emotional support throughout their children's formative years. Having risk-averse, poor risk-taker, and excessive parental monitoring and safety behaviours is thought to contribute directly to the development of depression. Emotional abuse, corporal punishment, and the development of a "socio traumatised personality," which may result in psychological distress, have a number of common characteristics. It is hypothesised that parental disappointment and judgement has negative effects on children's ability to regulate their emotions, children's sense of self-worth and competence, and children's beliefs and attributions about the social environment, all of which contribute to increased suffering.

Findings from previous studies indicate that rejection and overprotection and anxiety disorders are precursorsors for generalised anxiety and generalised separatism, respectively; these outcomes can manifest as depression and isolation, respectively, as raised children attempt to connect with others due to constant anxiety around attachment. Researchers are of the opinion that parents who raise their children in an unloving and controlling manner cause their children's self-efficacy to suffer, which in turn leads to the development of anxiety and depression in the youngsters.

Parenting Style And Delinquency

The Latin root for delinquency is 'delinquere,' which is composed of the prefix 'de' meaning 'away' and the root 'linquere' meaning 'to leave' or 'to forsake. The original meaning of the word "delinquency" related to youngsters whose parents had left them to fend for themselves. Adolescent delinquency might have its roots in childhood behavioral issues. Infractions of rules and acts of violence such as theft, assault, and vandalism are all possible examples. After kids have reached high levels of antisocial conduct, they are less likely to return to lower levels of antisocial behavior. First, Hirschi (1969) proposed a criminological theory in which attachment is seen as an emotive relationship through which infants acquire customary rules of society. According to Hirschi, families with strong emotional links will have lower rates of juvenile delinquency because children who are linked to their parents are more likely to care about their parents' normative expectations, which in turn shield them from acting on their own delinquent tendencies. Parental authority is exerted indirectly via a child's attachment quality, which promotes more traditional conduct. For a lifetime of participation in property crimes, kindergarten-level physical violence was the sole reliable predictor. Acts or omissions that violate recognized moral norms constitute delinquency and are thus unacceptable in any community. Juvenile delinquency is defined as involvement in criminal activity by teenagers, whereas delinquency is used to describe anybody who commits an offense. In this context, "juvenile" refers to a minor who has committed a crime. A juvenile is a minor who has not reached the legal age of majority in his or her home country, does not look or behave like an adult, and may be held legally responsible for their unlawful behavior. Both responsiveness and demanding nests are lacking in the parenting style that might be described as negligent or uninvolved. Attachment to mothers was shown to be more significant for the development of delinquency in females, whereas attachment to dads was found to be more crucial for the development of delinquency in boys. The parents seldom ever keep an eye on their children or attempt to exert control or discipline on them. Teenagers that come from these kinds of homes often exhibit a wide variety of externalising behaviours, such as delinquent activities, drug abuse, and other related issues .One of the most pressing issues of our day is juvenile delinquency. The parenting style of an adolescent is heavily influenced by his or her parents. Studies confirm that strict parenting encourages delinquent habits and is a contributing factor in the development of antisocial conduct. While paternal psychopathology was found to be positively associated with offspring antisocial behavior only through the mediator role of parenting style, maternal psychopathology was found to be positively associated with antisocial behavior in children either directly or partially by parenting style. These connections were not affected in any way by the child's sexuality. The way in which parents with mental health issues raise their children might be a focus for the prevention and intervention of antisocial conduct in the children of such parents. The way parents raise their children may be a major contributor to the development of behavioural issues.

Ruchkin et al. (2000) noted, however, that parenting styles are merely a piece of a much larger system, and hence they should not be used in isolation to predict future behavioural difficulties. Adolescents may become more antisocial if their parents exercise cold, emotionless control over them, but no problems will arise if such control seems rational and is carried out in a loving, pleasant setting. Many studies have shown that young people whose parents used authoritarian or neglectful parenting approaches were more likely to experiment with these vices themselves. Parent as a potential offender-inducing family member. Drug-abusing parents, neglectful parents, a lack of positive reinforcement, physical abuse of children, a history of criminal conduct in the family, a large family, and other similar factors have all been linked to increased risk of antisocial behavior in children. A youngster brought up in this kind of household may be less able to recognize antisocial conduct in others. Parents may reassure their kid by creating an attachment environment in their interactions with the child, which includes providing comfort via nurturing, monitoring, and psychological control. In order to reduce juvenile delinquency, it is increasingly important to foster a sense of attachment in children, since attachment is a kind of contact that is employed often in social, therapeutic, developmental, and educational contexts. Having parents who are too easygoing was also linked to more teens smoking and drinking. It has also been shown that various parenting methods have varying associations with their children's dangerous conduct. One definition of parental partiality is prioritizing one kid above another (Yahav, 2006). Favorite kid receives their parents' undivided attention, affection, and praise. While making their selection, parents often look for a kid that has a skill or hobby that piques their interest. The youngster may have feelings of specialness and grandeur, but also remorse at the expense of his or her siblings. The rejected children may band together to take revenge on their favorite sibling. The favored kid may worry excessively about living up to the parents' expectations and feeling guilty for receiving special treatment while the siblings go without. The siblings' feelings of rejection and unappreciation by their parents might cause lasting emotional trauma. In this case, the answer relies on whether or not the parenting style was evaluated by the teenager, highlighting the need to take into account perspectives from both generations. Several studies confirm the beneficial effects of an authoritative parenting style on teenagers' growth and development. Adolescents are less likely to engage in delinquent or dangerous conduct when their parents keep a close eye on them and make sure they are exposed to beneficial activities (Wargo, 2007). Adolescents benefit from a loving but strong parenting style that sets limits and boundaries that are appropriate for their age group. Adolescence, identity development, and the mental health of adolescents were discussed in this chapter. Parenting methods and their categorization were also covered, as were the early and late phases of adolescence. Few studies have been conducted on the topic of gender variations in the relationship between attachment and criminal behavior, and those that have been done have produced conflicting results. Although some research found higher impacts of attachment in females, others came to the conclusion that males place a greater emphasis on the importance of the family relationship. It was shown that men were more susceptible to the negative impacts of family stress and the quality of parental caring than girls were. The lack of a stable bond was shown to have a much stronger correlation with boys' externalizing behavior than it did with girls' samples (Fearon et al. 2010).

Adolescents whose parents are emotionally distant, uncaring, and contemptuous are more likely to engage in antisocial conduct themselves. Evidence suggests that teenage emotional and behavioural difficulties might be influenced by attachment insecurity. A child's susceptibility to emotional and behavioural issues increases in proportion to the degree to which they exhibit insecure attachment. This fits the pattern shown in studies that link attachment instability to both internalising and externalising problems in children at different ages (Herrenkohl, et, al 2011).

The way in which parents choose to raise and care for their children has a direct bearing on the likelihood of their offspring being involved in criminal activity. Extreme control, stringent limits, harsh and discordant punishment, and a lack of emotional support are hallmarks of the authoritarian approach to parenting. Aggression, emotional deregulation, and other poor behavioural outcomes are linked to an authoritarian parenting style. Between the ages of 13 and 18, when persons are called teenagers, delinquent conduct is one of the most distressing issues that might arise. It has been suggested that, as a result of globalisation, crimes are getting more brutal in their execution. The importance of studying juvenile delinquency and assessing the impact of parenting styles as a root cause of this conduct has grown as the issue has become a societal concern. A child's family, as a socio-cultural and economic unit, plays a pivotal role in shaping not just the child's everyday actions but also their future personalities. According to Talib, et, al (2011), a child's family is a socio-cultural economic structure that significantly affects not only the child's conduct but also the child's character development. As a result, parents' lack of knowledge might have negative consequences, such as the development of behavioural issues in their children. As a result, parents' lack of knowledge might have negative consequences, such as the development of behavioural issues in their children. Adolescent delinquency is strongly linked to parents' authoritarian parenting styles and often has severe consequences (Kerr, Stattin & Ozdemir, 2012). It is believed that delinquent conduct results from the combination of a child's innate tendencies and environmental triggers. A child's family, parenting style, school environment, peer group, IQ, socioeconomic level, and emotional maturity may all have an impact on whether or not he or she is predisposed to delinquency. When a youngster has a propensity for delinquency, he or she may actively seek out situations that would bring out their worst tendencies. Delinquency proneness describes the possibility that a teen may engage in criminal behavior.

According to the findings of academic studies (Glueck & Glueck, 2013), one of the primary factors that contributes to a child's development towards a life of criminal behaviour is the impact of his or her family. There are many causes of neglectful parenting, such as parents putting themselves first, a lack of parental encouragement, financial difficulties, a lack of social support, and even drug abuse. Neglected children learn to internalise the message that they are less important to their parents than other priorities. This kind of upbringing encourages children to want to be self-sufficient, which might lead to their acting older than they are. Literature suggests that permissive parenting involves politeness; however, in this instance, the term politeness is better suited to be defined under the heading of authoritative parenting. This is because, in permissive parenting, parents are not involved in the process of developing their children's characters. Parents that are permissive let their children to actively engage in activities without being worried about what such activities may bring about (Bernardo, 2014). Parents and their offspring often act in opposite ways. When children stop engaging socially, they emotionally retreat. Relationships later in life are also impacted by this attachment disorder. One theory on why some kids act out is because they don't have a secure connection to their parents. A thorough study of the association between attachment and criminality has not yet been done, despite the fact that numerous empirical researches have revealed evidence that weak connection to parents increases the probability of delinquent behavior. Having a firm grasp of the correlation between secure attachment and juvenile delinquency across sexes and ages would be useful in designing and refining effective intervention strategies.

The adolescent may have a history of truancy and criminal behaviour. It is a commonly held belief that parenting styles are the primary cause of delinquent conduct in the majority of children and adolescents. When teenagers are subjected to factors such as anger and blame, they are more likely to engage in delinquent conduct. These factors include a lack of intimacy, lack of direction, lack of parental participation, lack of parental connection, and lack of parental involvement. So, it would not be incorrect to argue that there is a considerable relationship between the parenting methods of an individual and the individual's propensity to participate in antisocial or aggressive conduct. In other words, a lack of engagement and contact on the part of parents leads to an increased risk of violent behaviour in adolescents, particularly in males (Brook et al, 2014). In most cases, a parent who neglects their children lacks respect for them and so causes them to feel rejected, angry and alone. Adolescents' conduct may be significantly influenced by their parents. Young men make up the vast majority of juvenile delinquents, and they are disproportionately responsible for committing violent and illegal acts such as rape, murder, and property offences. As the world becomes more interconnected, statistics show that violent crimes are also growing more common (Siegel & Welsh, 2014). Juvenile delinquency has become a serious societal issue, making it crucial to examine the issue and assess the impact of parenting methods as potential root causes of the problem. An individual's parenting style has a significant impact on their child's risk for delinquency (Coste, 2015). More often than not, parents are held accountable for their children's illegal or delinquent actions. Some legal systems even hold parents legally responsible for their children's rude or criminal behaviour. According to the research that was looked at, an authoritarian parenting style is the one that is most suited for young children in order to protect them from developing a criminal mindset.

For instance, according to the research that was looked at, an authoritarian parent is one that exercises strict control over their children, instills a sense of discipline in them, and maintains the belief that a kid ought to behave in a manner that is congruent with ethical standards. This is especially the case as a result of the increased worry among parents over the authoritarian parenting style that is prevalent in conventional family structures. The autonomy of their offspring and the bond between the parent and kid are both restricted when seen from this point of view. Children may be predicted to have a favourable development if they have a safe and high-quality connection to their parents. This positive development can include an exceptional ability to adjust to campus life, confidence in interpersonal relationships, and the pursuit of vocational objectives. On the other hand, insecurities and a poor quality of connection to one's parents are highly connected with depressive and anxious states in adolescents, as well as suicidal tendencies, illegal conduct, substance misuse, and criminal activity. (Chen, et, al, 2017). Those who experience unfavourable parent-child connections in early infancy are more likely to develop pessimistic worldviews, believe that other people are untrustworthy and dangerous, and struggle to love and accept themselves. As a result, kids may experience issues such as homelessness, slowed moral development, aggression, and antisocial tendencies (Khoury, et, al, 2020).

CHAPTER-4

CONCLUSION

To be a parent is the most satisfying job in the world. Raising a healthy, successful, and loving kid is the greatest source of pride and happiness a parent can have. Parents are the most influential people in a child's life since they are the major socializers. It is difficult to bring up a kid who will grow up to be happy and successful. The best methods for doing this are unknown. Examining the impact of various parenting techniques on a child's sense of self-worth is one approach to this problem. It's hard to claim with certainty that any one of the four primary parenting styles—authoritarian, authoritative, permissive, and neglectful—is ideal for every child. The Ramayana and the Mahabharata, two of India's most well-known epics, both include stories of a child's undying love and devotion for his or her parents and traditional Hindu traditions place an emphasis on maintaining close family connections as one grows older (Larson, 2003). Parents are expected to take initiative, participate actively, and provide support. The presence of unfavorable conditions at home has the potential to have an impact on academic achievement. When parents get disenchanted with the schooling of their children, they are less likely to be aware of how their children are doing in school. Parenting takes far longer in Indian culture, and children rely on their parents for a longer period of time. Raising kids in an authoritative household was more effective than either a permissive or authoritative one in developing confident adults. Hence, it is the responsibility of family counselors to advise new parents on how to best foster their children's emotional, psychological, and social growth. Adolescents from various cultural backgrounds and communities have varying effects from parental styles and disciplinary practices. Recent years have seen significant progress in our knowledge of how parenting practices and philosophies affect the mental and behavioural health of adolescents. Parental influence throughout adolescence continues to effect behaviours into adulthood, making empirical study concentrating on the links between parenting and teenage outcomes relevant. It's no secret that parents have a substantial influence on their children's mental health, a fundamental factor in their development. Parent-child spatial problem-solving tasks (such as joint block building, puzzle tasks, or origami activities) have been studied for their potential to reveal the quality of parental learning stimulation in early childhood, with better general learning support during these spatial activities being predictive of later math and overall school achievement.

One of the most significant determinants of mental health is the quality of one's relationships, including those between parents and their children. Poor mental health may be a result of poor parenting, which includes poor parent-child communication and engagement. Simply said, a parent's parenting style is how they interact with one another and their children. In addition to reducing the prevalence of mental diseases, authoritative parenting has also been shown to improve mental health. Moreover, it mitigates the harmful effects of stress on health, serves as a predictor of academic performance, and is linked to better levels of education attainment, all of which are beneficial to the development of healthy adolescents. In reality, when someone's mental health is poor, they are less able to carry out their responsibilities, which slow down the process and have negative knock-on effects. Parental authority, whether proposed or delivered in the form of a lecture, is intolerable to adolescents. Self-confidence and the hope for a brighter tomorrow are products of people's psychological development. The world is more stable when parents are able to reproduce healthy, whole human beings. You can teach your kids to be influential people by being a prepared and caring parent. Adolescence is a time when a kid must come to grips with his or her own identity; therefore it is especially important for parents to know that they are using rigorous yet loving parenting approaches and not using a heavy hand on their children. If parents have more faith in their child's skills, this might have a positive effect on the child's academic performance.

Parents play a big part in a teen's quest for independence and self-identity. Successful parents instilled in their kids a sense of stability that motivates them to take initiative and work for independence. Ideally, parents would want to assist their adolescents in developing their identities and allow them to try out new ideas and behaviours during the period of life known as adolescence, when an individual tends to be more concerned with them rather than being psychologically dependent on family. The development of identity and independence in this environment involves both the teenager and his parent as part of a joint and interdependent process. To ensure that no parent is left out of the connection, parents cooperate to care for and discipline their children. The teenager might then begin to articulate his own perspectives after gaining clarity about his connections to others. They will be aware of and accountable for their own thoughts and actions, as well as the thoughts and actions of others. Only when parents and children have a quality connection can adolescents develop social competence. When surrounded by their peers, kids gain self-assurance and a sense of social responsibility. Otherwise, the youth will lose all of these to a non qualitative connection. This will have a detrimental impact on their capacity to establish a sense of self and autonomy. The research is unequivocal in demonstrating that the quality of the bond that exists between adolescents and their parents continues to be an important factor in determining health throughout all stages of development. It is essential that practitioners working in mental health, along with those working in other areas of health and education, have understanding of adolescent development and the significance of adolescent-parent attachment. Adolescents may experience identity crisis if their parents model undesirable behaviours and attitudes. It might even cause teenagers to grow up with complexes. Being too authoritative may also have a negative impact on teenagers' mental health, which can impede their development of a healthy sense of self. Hence, it is recommended that all parents of teenagers employ appropriate parenting approaches and helps their children develop into physically and psychologically healthy adults. There is a substantial and significant beneficial connection between the manner in which a child is raised and their level of self-esteem. A greater level of self-esteem is associated with having parents who are authoritative. Children who experience a parenting style that is both authoritarian and lenient tend to have lower levels of self-esteem. Adolescents whose parents exhibit an authoritarian parenting style are more likely to engage in antisocial behaviour because of the extreme discipline they are subjected to. To this end, authoritative parenting entails keeping a close check on one's offspring and making an effort to comprehend their point of view. When it comes to their children's growth, authoritarian parents sometimes exert too much control, which is seen adversely by their offspring. There are four main ways in which children experience their parents' rejection: when they are cold and unaffectionate; when they are hostile and aggressive; when they are indifferent and neglectful; and when there are no clear behavioral indicators of parental rejection but the children still feel rejected. Perceived parental rejection is significantly linked to overall adolescent maladjustment, as shown by many studies. A child's ability to control his or her emotions, to form a healthy sense of self-worth and competence, and to form accurate beliefs and attributions about the external environment are all thought to be negatively impacted by parental rejection and criticism, leading to an increase in the child's anxiety levels.

Adolescent delinquency is mostly fueled by a variety of variables, but neglect is a particularly potent one. The lack of parental supervision might lead to a rise in antisocial behavior in youngsters. Neglecting to handle delinquent conduct when it is brought to attention is an example of a lack of parental control. It's possible that parents who are frightened of upsetting their kids or who see their kids' transgressions as minor and hence never discipline them can exhibit such behavior. They may have a hard time making friends and controlling their emotions, but kids raised by these sorts of parents adore their parents. In addition, these actions put kids at risk for engaging in frequent school fights or adopting delinquent habits as a means of gaining social acceptance. When a child's delinquent conduct seems to be a problem, the attachment style of the child's parents is a crucial factor to consider. Many parents in the past struggled to form strong bonds with their children because they had to work long hours to meet their financial obligations. Low income made parents less likely to invest time in strengthening family bonds. Some parents have come to understand the need of fostering close relationships with their children in order to prevent the development of antisocial behaviors. Ineffective parenting has been connected by several thinkers to juvenile delinquency. Children raised in such environments often have attachment insecurities and feel alone in times of difficulty.

In conclusion, it is recommended that parents focus more importance on the ways they may interact with their children and utilize this time to have them better prepare for careers. The relevance of children should be communicated to the local community and the techniques of interaction to them should be made known via mass media and family preparedness. If you want your kids to grow up to be good people, you need to make sure you and them have a good connection at home and at school. Children's lives, from conception through early development, are profoundly shaped by their parents. Teenagers spend a lot of time at home, thus parental influences, as well as the family's own beliefs and expectations, may have significant effects on their development. The detrimental impact on a kid's life of a parent's parenting style increases as the degree to which the youngster is subjected to severe or lavish treatment increases. Parents' caring, empathetic, and less judgemental attitudes are the most crucial elements in raising healthy adolescents.

CHAPTER-5

EDUCATIONAL IMPLICATIONS AND RECOMMENDATION

In the current context, teenagers' academic achievements play a crucial part in molding their character and conduct. High school students feel more pressure to succeed in an increasingly competitive academic environment. Reducing such stress and increasing adolescents' efficiency in bettering their academic performance are crucial roles played by parental connection, student involvement, and buoyancy. Anyone involved in education (parents, educators, guidance counselors, and administrators) may draw direct conclusions from the findings. Counselors and parents should be aware of the significance that academic achievement has in the lives of adolescents. Thus, they may work with faculty and management to develop and execute strategies designed to improve student achievement in the classroom. Students will do better in school if their parents and teachers are able to communicate openly and work together to aid them. As a result, parents should encourage and demonstrate connection to their children in order to help them succeed academically and so mitigate any associated risks. If students are not adequately prepared for the stress and psychological symptoms to which they may be exposed due to their academic achievement, then the time, money, and human resources spent in their education will be for nothing. Education authorities are urged to provide instructors with additional training that would enable them to assist kids see the difference between their own value and academic achievement, encourage a growth mindset in the face of academic failure, foster a cooperative environment, and more. On top of that, there are a plethora of abilities that may lessen their psychological risk factors, promoting a feeling of control by giving pupils the right objectives and tasks and focusing their attention on the right ways to get high grades. This book suggests that parental connection does not act as a moderator between a child's academic success and their level of psychological risk, engagement, and buoyancy in the classroom. It was concluded that effective practices and pedagogies improve student outcomes by helping students develop their skills, giving them chances to achieve their full potential, and giving them regular, timely feedback on their progress. Hence, it would be crucial to take into account learning styles and tempos, as well as a variety of skills, concrete methods for enhancing education, and an evaluation designed to encourage student participation. It has also been shown that pupils have a positive attitude about their academic careers. Hence, it is crucial for them to comprehend the academic challenges they experience, the most important of which is the adaptive means by which adolescents should comprehend. Therefore, effective strategies to protect youth from the various factors are required, and teachers can assist students in improving their academic performance by assisting them in comprehending lessons, performing tasks based on daily tasks, planning for effective learning, increasing their efforts to comprehend assignments, and understanding the factors for academic success and failure.

Recommendation

Humans aren't the only creatures on Earth that experience the phenomena of parenting. Personal and social changes, environmental pressures, the company of peers and family, and the pressure to adapt academically are all risk factors in a child's development, and a parent's behaviour may have a significant impact on how those risks play out. The parent-child connection benefits from, and is facilitated by, the positivity of the parent's approach and outlook. Anyone interested in raising public consciousness regarding the impact parents have on their teenage children's development should read this book. Children learn both directly and indirectly from their parents, so it's important for them to pay attention to and spend time with them. Both parents and children should have easy access to counseling and therapy services to assist them work through their issues. Children will feel more secure if they are cared for and supported by their parents. It is important for parents to foster an atmosphere at home that encourages their children's growth of self-assurance, since this will help them feel more at ease in the wider world, allowing them to focus more easily and, in turn, improve their academic performance. The best way to prevent a youngster from feeling ignored is for parents to be attentive to his or her needs. They may be unable to focus on their schoolwork because they feel ignored, which will affect their grades.

Parents can't know everything, and they may benefit from training themselves. This might improve their communication, allow them to better understand their children's personalities, and encourage them to work together to find solutions to any issues that arise. This is of paramount significance while youngsters are in their adolescent years. Parents worry about their children's well-being and safety, thus they should be adaptable and open to new ideas. They believe that providing a nurturing home and plenty of positive reinforcements are more effective than harsh discipline when it comes to raising a responsible, independent youngster. This research shows how important it is to take into account cultural variations when analysing parenting styles. Hence, there should be further longitudinal and cultural research. Qualitative research on the effects of parenting on teenagers is needed. Relationships between parents and offspring are complex and mutually influential. Parents, educators, and mental health experts all need to give parenting styles greater consideration, and society has to take action to raise parents' awareness of the issue. It's important for parents to put themselves in their teenage children's shoes. They should not have lofty expectations of the youngster either. Their potential and level of ability should inform your expectations. The role of the educator is to foster a robust and optimistic outlook on life in the young people under their care. In order for students to develop into mentally healthy and effective members of society who can work for both their own and their country's well-being, educators have a duty to implement socially acceptable practices to alleviate students' anxiety, fear, despair, and dissatisfaction. Policymakers in the fields of school counseling and psychology should develop programmes that specifically reach out to parents in order to help them gain insight into their own parenting practices, which might lead to early intervention mental health treatment. To evaluate whether or not a couple's parenting approaches are consistent, researchers should seek out people who reside with both parents. This is crucial because researchers need to include both the mother and the father when evaluating whether or not there is consistency in their parenting. To help students succeed academically, educational administrators should tailor the curriculum to their requirements. Since children come from diverse households, some are shy, others are hyperactive, and teachers should utilize varied ways. .In today's world, it's crucial for parents to be self-aware in regards to their parenting style. It's true that other institutions in society have assumed many of the roles traditionally played by families, but ultimately its parents who have the most influence on their children's development as social beings. So, the way they raise their children has far-reaching effects on the world at large. There is a robust correlation between an authoritative parenting style and normal teenage growth. The freedom to experiment with independence, within reasonable bounds, is made possible by a firm structure for young people. So, if they want their children to grow up healthy and powerful, parents should adopt an authoritative approach. Both authoritarian and permissive parents may improve their parenting styles by taking a step back and reevaluating their methods. The parental roles and obligations need to be reevaluated (mother and father). They should use these methods to give kids a voice in discussions about right and wrong. Exchanges of words between parents and children may do wonders for the latter's sense of self and the former's capacity for empathy. While authoritarian parenting methods, as well as negligent and permissive parenting styles, were shown to link adversely with the students' levels of self-esteem, it is advised that parents exercise greater authority in their parenting. The parents need to enable the children to make their own personal choices, after which they ought to constructively endorse or condemn the decisions via communication that goes in both directions. It is very essential that parents have an attitude that is very supportive and encouraging towards their children. In order for their children to grow up emotionally healthy, parents should pay close attention to them and provide guidance or counseling. Their youngsters are vulnerable and should not be subjected to any criticism or criticism from others. They shouldn't feel pressured to do well on the test. Parents may work on improving their children's study habits by enacting constructive intervention strategies. It is imperative that the nation's policymakers take reformatory steps to develop the appropriate institutional atmosphere and the practices being followed in schools throughout the country in order to improve students' mental health. By educating parents about the pros and cons of various parenting approaches, we may encourage them to choose strategies that will have a favorable impact on their children's development. It sheds light on the ways in which different parenting methods affect teenagers' emotional quotient. Parents should take an interest in their children's academic progress and extracurricular activities. The objective is for them to take greater responsibility for their studies. In order to help their children succeed in school, parents need be familiar with the ideas of reinforcement and motivation and use them constructively. There are instances when parents should encourage their children to take the initiative. The youngster should be given a voice in certain choices but should always be led by their parents.

Parents should praise their children more and appreciate their accomplishments, avoid harmful criticism and outright condemnation in the presence of their children's contemporaries, and promote the good characteristics in their children rather than focusing on their children's shortcomings. Parents should steer clear of any types of put-down jokes and mockery directed at their children since they are major contributors to youngsters having poor self-esteem. For kids to have higher levels of self-esteem, it is suggested that school counsellors implement several self-esteem development programmes. For the sake of the students' growth, it is incumbent upon them to provide a secure setting. Teens should learn from their counsellors about adjusting to their parents' parenting methods, whether those approaches are different from their own or ones they've embraced themselves. The counsellor may assist boost kids' self-esteem and emotional intelligence by posting inspirational statements and passages on classroom bulletin boards. Parents have a crucial role in helping their children develop their talents and skills. It is ideal for parents and children to have a tight, trusting connection based on mutual understanding. Thus, it is suggested that the proper methods of interaction between parents and children be given more weight, and that parents acquaint their children with the roles of businesses in society and the necessity of employment in legitimate businesses, and that this crucial matter be given more emphasis through the media and family training classes. Parents should trust their kids and let them supervise themselves. Academic assignments may boost academic self-efficacy and emotional management. Be cognizant of cultural differences and create educational policy that promotes academic success. Adolescents may be deterred from criminal behaviour and the company of lawbreakers by their parents' consistent involvement with their offspring. Having positive relationships with their parents is an important factor in preventing juvenile delinquency. This book is a great resource for learning how to execute psychological therapies with the goal of improving parent-child relationships. Particularly, supporting parents with insecure attachment to increase their emotional control may be a way to boost their parenting abilities and better the parent-child bond.

Counselors in schools should provide regular emotional coaching. This entails assisting parents in relating to their children by identifying, recognising, and affirming the emotions and sentiments that may be causing the disruptive behaviour rather than discarding them. If a child gives up at the first sight of difficulty, it may be because they don't have the safety net they need to try again. If educators really want to see their students succeed academically, they need to model stability for them. Policymakers also need to come up with a system to record attachment's significance in official records. Parents need reliable knowledge about the significant neurocognitive, social, and emotional changes that take place throughout adolescence, as well as the significance of their continuous sensitivity and attunement to their child's needs during this time period. They need to have a clear idea of what the future holds for them in terms of their connection with their kid, as well as the best way to handle the transition into adulthood. Many parents see the rise in hostility between their children and them that often happens throughout the teenage years as their kid's way of rejecting them personally along with the connection and their significance to the youngster. In order to ensure their children have the best possible future, parents should spend quality time with them, adopt a family-focused philosophy, encourage their children to take responsibility for their own well-being, inspire them, boost their self-esteem, provide them with moral support, etc. People in today's materialistic world are so preoccupied with making ends meet that they have trouble spending enough quality time with their children, which may lead to a variety of personality and behavioural flaws. Considering the attachment bond with parents as a goal of intervention when working with juvenile offenders or at-risk youngsters is important. These programs should also work to strengthen parental disciplinary practices, since these issues often coexist with insecure attachment and weak relationships to children.

It was discovered that teachers were the only professionals working in the school; as a result, students did not have access to the support of other professionals who could assist them in overcoming their personal and familial issues, which had a negative impact on both their education and their personal lives. Because of the way things were at the school, there has to be a revision made to the rules on the services that are required to be offered to children while they are there. Not only should school serve as a hub for educational opportunities, but it should also be a location that places a major emphasis on the overall growth and development of its pupils.

References

- Allen, J. P, Porter, M., McFarland, C, McElhaney, K. B. & Marsh, P. (2007). The relation of attachment security to adolescents' paternal and peer relationships, depression, and externalizing behavior. Child Development, 78, 1222 – 1239.

- Amy, M., (2019). 4 Types of Parenting Styles and Their Effects on Kids. Child Development. Updated on July 12, 2019 [4] Arigabu,

- Arafat, A. (2022). Parenting Style and Suicidal Behavior: A Focused Review. Hindawi Mental Illness.

- B. R. Sahithya, S. M. Manohari, and R. Vijaya, "Parenting styles and its impact on children – a cross cultural review with a focus on India," *Mental Health, Religion & Culture*, vol. 22, no. 4, pp. 357–383, 2019.

- Bernardo, L. L. A. (2014). *The influence of parenting styles on* the *family relationships of lesbians and gay men*. Retrieved from-

  http://udr.slu.edu.ph:8080/jspui/handle/123456789/269

- Bornstein, M. H. (2001). Parenting: Science and practice. Parenting, 1(1-2), 1-4.
- Bowlby J. *Attachment and Loss: Volume 2. Separation.* New York: Basic Books; 1973. [Google Scholar]
- Bradley H. R., Corwyn F. R. (2002) Socioeconomic Status and Child Development. Annual Review of Psychology, Vol. 53, pp. 371-399.
- Brook, D. W., Brook, J. S., Rosen, Z., De la Rosa, M., Montoya, I. D., & Whiteman, M. (2014). Early risk factors for violence in Colombian adolescents. *American Journal of Psychiatry 160*(8), 1470-1478.
- Chen, W. *et al.* Perceived social support and self-esteem as mediators of the relationship between parental attachment and life satisfaction among Chinese adolescents. *Pers. Individ. Differ.* **108**, 98–102 (2017).
- Clark, K. E and Ladd, G. W. (2000). Connectedness and autonomy support in parent- child relationships: Links to children's socioemotional orientation and peer relationship. Developmental Psychology, 36, 485–498

- Coste, B. (2015). Positive parenting: Practicle advice and deep insights. Retrieved from http://www.positive-parenting-ally. com/3-parenting-styles.html

- Deci, E. L., & Ryan, R. M. (1985). Intrinsic motivation and self-determination in human behavior. New York: Plenum Press.

- Deshpande, A., Chhabriya, M. (2013). Parenting Styles and its Effects on Adolescents' SelfEsteem. vol 2.0 (2). 163–176.

- Diniz, E., Brandao, T., Monteiro, L., and Veríssimo, M. (2021). Father involvement during early childhood: a systematic review of the literature. *J. Fam. Theory Rev.* 13, 77–99.

- Dishion TJ, McMahon RJ. *Clinical Child and Family Psychology Review.* 1998:61-75. doi:10.1023/a:1021800432380

- Fearon RP, Bakermans-Kranenburg MJ, IJzendoorn a M H v, Lapsley A-M, Roisman GI. The significance of insecure attachment and disorganization in the development of children's externalizing behavior: a meta-analytic study. *Child Development.* 2010;81(2):435–456

❖ Fisher, R.L. (1974). Media Review: Books: Attachment and Loss, Separation: Anxiety and Anger. Exceptional Children, 41(1):61-62.

❖ Fonte, B. A. (2009). Relationship between parenting style, emotional intelligene and self-esteem. Retrieved October 6, 2009, from http://hdl.handle.net/10090/7271.

❖ Garcia, Q.P. & Santiago, A.B. (2017). Parenting styles as correlates to self-esteem of underprivileged adolescents: basis for a proposed parenting skills program. International Journal of Advanced Education and Research. 2 (5), 27- 35.

❖ George, C., and Solomon, J. (1999). "Attachment and caregiving: the caregiving behavioral system," in *Handbook of attachment: Theory, research, and clinical applications*, eds J. Cassidy and P. Shaver (New York, NY: Guilford Press).

❖ Gilmour, H. (2014). Positive mental health and mental illness. Health Report, 25(9), 3–9

- Glueck, S., & Glueck, E. (2013). Family environment and delinquency. New York: Routledge.

- Hesari, N., & Hejazi, E (2011). The Mediating Role of Self Esteem in the Relationship Between the Authoritative Parenting Style and Aggression. Procedia-Social and Behavioral Sciences. 30:1724-1730.

- Hirschi, T. (1969). *Causes of delinquency*. Berkeley: University of California Press.

- Hong, O., Long, C., & Abdull Rahman, R. (2015). An Analysis on the Relationship between Parenting Styles and Self Esteem of Students of a University in Malaysia: A Case Study. Mediterranean Journal Of Social Sciences, 6 (4), 300. Retrieved from http://www.mcser.org/journal/index.php/mjss/article/view/7291

- Illing, V., Tasca, G. A., Balfour, L., & Bissada, H. (2010). Attachment insecurity predicts eating disorder symptoms and treatment outcomes in a clinical sample of women. The Journal of Nervous and Mental Disease, 198(9), 653-659. https://doi.org/10.1097/NMD.0b013e3181ef34b2

- Jones, J., Cassidy, J., and Shaver, P. (2015). Parents' self-reported attachment styles: A review of links with parenting behaviors, emotions, and cognitions. *Pers. Soc. Psychol. Rev.* 1, 44–76. doi: 10.1177/1088868314541858

- Joshi, H. L., Sharma, M., & Mehra, R. K. (2009). Depression among adolescents: Role of self efficacy and parenting style. Journal of Psychology & Mental Health, Vol. 16, 13- 17.

- Kawamoto, T. (2020). The moderating role of attachment style on the relationship between self-concept clarity and self-esteem. *Personality and Individual Differences*, *152*, 109604.

- Kerr, M., Stattin, H., & Ozdemir, M. (2012). Perceived parenting style and adolescent adjustment: Revisiting directions of effects and the role of parental knowledge. *Developmental Psychology, 48*(6), 1540.

- Khoury, J. E., Rajamani, M., Bureau, J.-F., Easterbrooks, M. & Lyons-Ruth, K. Aspects of parent–child interaction from infancy to late adolescence are associated with severity of childhood maltreatment through age 18. *Int. J. Environ. Res. Public Health* **17**, 3749 (2020).

- Kumar, R. & Fernandez D., (2017). An Empirical Study of Assertiveness Among Business Students: A Case Study of Nizwa College of Technology, Sultanate of Oman. European Journal of Business and Management. www.iiste.org ISSN 2222-1905 (Paper) ISSN 2222-2839 (Online), 9,2.

- Labovit, B. (2015).Perceived Parenting Styles and their Impact on Depressive Symptoms in Adolescent 15-18 Years Old. Journal of Educational and Social Rcscarch, 5 (1), 171-176. doi:10.5901/jesr.2015.v5n1p171

- Larson, R.E. E. D., Verma, S. U. M. A. N., & Dworkin, J. (2003). Adolescence without family disengagement: The daily family lives of Indian middle-class teenagers: Theory, research and applications. In Cross-cultural perspectives in human development: Theory, research and applications. Sage

- Li, M., Chen, X., Gong, H., Ji, W., Wang, W., Liang, S., & Kong, A. (2021). The predictive effect of parental adult attachment on parent–adolescent attachment: The mediating role of harsh parenting. *Frontiers in Psychology*, *12*, 3380

- Lightfoot, C., Cole, M & Cole, S. (2009). The development of children. New York: Worth Publishers.

- Liu Y.L. Parental/maternal attachment, peer support, social expectations of peer interaction, and depressive symptoms. Adolescence 2006 41 705 21

- Liu, X., Zhao, L., and Su, Y. S. (2022). Impact of parents' attitudes on learning ineffectiveness: the mediating role of parental self-efficacy. *Int. J. Environ. Res. Public Health* 19:615. doi: 10.3390/ijerph19010615

- Martinez, I., and Garcia, J, (2008): Internalization of values and self-esteem among Brazilian teenagers from authoritative, indulgent, authoritarian, and neglectful homes. Family Therapy, Journal of Personality and Social Psychology, 35(1), 2008, 43-59.

- Milu, M. A. & Fathima, M.A.(2015). Perceived maternal parenting styles and self-esteem among adolescents. Indian Journal of Applied Research. 5(8). 504-506

- Moore, O. (2011). *Influence of parental involvement on the academic achievement of adolescents*. Paper presented at the Paper Presented at the Annual Conference of the American Psychological Association, Washington D.C.

- Mulyadi, S., Rahardjo, W., & Basuki, A.H. (2016). The role of parent-child relationship, self-esteem, academic self-efficacy to academic stress. Procedia-Social and Behavioral Sciences, 217: 603-608.

- Nijhof, K. S., C., R., & Engels, M. E. (2007). Parenting styles, coping strategies and the expression of homesickness. *Journal of Adolescence, 30*(5), 709-720.

- Nikoogoftar, M &Seghatoleslam, S. (2015).The Role of Parenting Styles in Predicting Adolescent Behavioural and Emotional Problems. Practice in Clinical Psychology, 3(1), 23-30.

- Okoli, PC., Ezeme, MS, Chime, PE., Ozougwu, AO., Ofojebe, CP., Edoka, AC., & Akpoke, VO (2020) The Correlate of Personality Traits and Parenting Styles with Relapse in Alcohol amongst Treated Alcoholic Patients. J Alcohol Drug Depend 8:329. doi: 10.35248/2329-6488.20.8.329

❖ Peng, J., Lu, H., Zhang, J. *et al.* Parental attachment and emotional intelligence mediates the effect of childhood maltreatment on callous-unemotional traits among incarcerated male adolescents. *Sci Rep* **12**, 21214 (2022). https://doi.org/10.1038/s41598-022-25285-0

❖ Priya, D., & Jaswanti, V. P. (2020). Relationship between parenting styles and emotional intelligence among late adolescents in Chennai. The International Journal of Indian Psychology ISSN 2348-5396 (Online) | ISSN: 2349-3429 (Print) Volume 8, Issue 2, AprilJune, 2020. https://doi.org/10.25215/0802.023

❖ R. S. Banstola, T. Ogino, and S. Inoue, "Impact of parents' knowledge about the development of self-esteem in adolescents and their parenting practice on the self-esteem and suicidal behavior of urban high school students in Nepal," *International Journal of Environmental Research and Public Health*, vol. 17, no. 17, p. 6039, 2020.

❖ Ran, Z. O. U., Zeb, S., Nisar, F., Yasmin, F., Poulova, P., and Haider, S. A. (2022). The impact of emotional intelligence on career decision-making difficulties and generalized self-efficacy among university students in china. *Psychol. Res. Behav. Manage.* 15:865. doi: 10.2147/PRBM.S358742

- Ruchkin VV, Eisemann M, Koposov RA, Hägglöf B. Family functioning, parental rearing and behavioural problems in delinquents. *Clin Psychol Psychother.* 2000; **7** (4) : 310 -9

- S. Y. Arafat, H. Akter, M. A. Islam, M. M. A. Shah, and R. Kabir, "Parenting: types, effects and cultural variation," *Asian Journal of Pediatric Research*, vol. 3, pp. 32–36, 2020.

- Sankar, R., Wani, A., & Indumathi, R. (2017), Mental Health among Adolescents, International Journal of Indian Psychology, 4, (3), doi:10.25215/0403.102

- Santrock, J. W. (1995). Adolescence.12th Edition, New York: McGraw Hill

- Schimmenti, A. *et al.* Traumatic experiences, alexithymia, and Internet addiction symptoms among late adolescents. A moderated mediation analysis. *Addict. Behav.* 64, 314–320 (2017).

- Segal, J., Glenn, M., & Robinson, L., (2019). *What is secure attachment and bonding? Understanding the different ways of bonding and communicating with your infant or child.* Retrieved August from www.helpguide.org.

❖ Sharma D. (2003) Childhood, family, and Sociological Changes in India. Oxford University Press, New Delhi, p. 21.

❖ Shaver, P., and Mikulincer, M. (2002). Attachment-related psychodynamics. *Attach. Hum. Dev.* 4, 133–161. doi: 10.1080/14616730210154171

❖ Shilpa, S.(2014). Association between perceived parenting styles and positive mental health among college students in the age group 18 to 24 years (Doctoral dissertation, SCTIMST).Thiruvananthapuram , Kerala

❖ Siegel, L., & Welsh, B. (2014). *Juvenile delinquency: Theory, practice, and law.* Stamford: Cengage Learning.

❖ Sigelman C. K. (1999) Lifespan Human Development, Third Edition. Brooks/Cole Publishing Company, p. 40

❖ Smart, D. & Sanson, A. (2003). Social competence in young adulthood, its nature & antecedents. Melbourne: Australian Institute of Family Studies.

- Song, C., Ge, S., Xue, J., and Yao, W. (2022). Physical exercise of primary and middle school students from the perspective of educational psychology and parents' entrepreneurship education. *Front. Psychol.* 12:777069. doi: 10.3389/fpsyg.2021.777069

- Sousa C, Herrenkohl TI, Moylan CA, Tajima EA, Kilka JB, Herrenkohl RC, Russo MJ. Longitudinal study on the effects of child abuse and children's exposure to domestic violence, parent child attachments and antisocial behavior in adolescence. J Interpers Viol. 2011;26(1):111–36.

- Speranza, A. M., Quintigliano, M., Lauriola, M., and Fortunato, A. (2020). P-CRS: A clinical scale to assess the parent-child relationship in infancy and early childhood. *Intern. J. Envir. Res. Public Health* 17:3458. doi: 10.3390/ijerph17103458

- Ştefan, C. A., and Avram, J. (2017). Investigating direct and indirect effects of attachment on internalizing and externalizing problems through emotion regulation in a cross-sectional study. *J. Child Fam. Stud.* 26, 2311–2323. doi: 10.1007/s10826-017-0723-7

- Szkody, E., Steele, E. H., & McKinney, C. (2021). Effects of Parenting Styles on Psychological Problems by Self Esteem and Gender Differences. *Journal of Family Issues*, *42*(9), 1931–1954.

- Talib, M. B. A., Abdullah, R., & Mansor, M. (2011). Relationship between parenting style and children's behavior problems. *Asian Social Science,* *7*(12), p195.

- Tazouti, Y., and Jarlégan, A. (2019). The mediating effects of parental self-efficacy and parental involvement on the link between family socioeconomic status and children's academic achievement. *J. Fam. Stud.* 25, 250–266.

- Tiwari (2013). Mental health status of adolescents in relation to perceived parental support. Journal of the Indian Academy of Applied Psychology. 39 (2), 213-221.

- Turner, L. A. (2009). The influence of parenting styles, Achievement motivation. *Journal of Student Development,* *5*(6), 337-346.

- Turner, L. A. (2009). The influence of parenting styles, Achievement motivation. *Journal of Student Development,* 5(6), 337-346.

- Vandeleur, C. L., Perrez, M., and Schoebi, D. (2007). Associations between measures of emotion and familial dynamics in normative families with adolescents. Swiss Journal of Psychology, 66(1), 5e16

- Vora, K. (2013). A Study of Perceived Parenting in Relation to Mental Health and Social Maturity among Adolescents. Ph.D. (Psy.) thesis, SNDT Women's University, Retrieved on 3.5.17 from shodhganga.inflibnet.ac.in/ handle/ 10603/45039

- Wargo, E. (2007). Adolescents and Risk: Helping young people make better choices. Research facts and findings, Act for Youth Centre for excellence. New York: University of Rochester,

- Yahav, R. (2006). The relationship between children's and adolescents' perceptions of parenting style and internal and external symptoms. University of Haifa.

❖ Yang, F., & Liang, N. (2008). A study on the influence of early experiences on adolescents' implicit self-esteem. Psychological Science (China), 31(3), 556-561.

❖ Yusup, N. & Ahmad, M. (2016). The Influence of Parents support and its relationship with students' achievement in English Education. International Conference on Education and Regional Development (ICERD 2016), "Cross-Cultural Education for Sustainable Regional Development" Bandung, Indonesia, 657 – 662.

❖ Zhang, R., Chen, J., Lei, W., Liang, X., & Liu, Z. (2019). The mediating effect of interpersonal relationship on loneliness and negative emotions of secondary nursing students. Chinese Journal of Health Psychology, 27(7):1100- 1104.

Made in the USA
Monee, IL
04 November 2026

67386134R10081